GROWING PHYSICIAN LEADERS

*Empowering Doctors
to Improve Our Healthcare*

MARK HERTLING, DBA

AdventHealth Press

AdventHealth

GROWING PHYSICIAN LEADERS

Copyright © 2016 Mark Hertling
Published by AdventHealth Press
605 Montgomery Road, Altamonte Springs, FL 32714

EXTENDING *the* HEALING MINISTRY *of* CHRIST

EDITOR-IN-CHIEF	Todd Chobotar
COLLABORATIVE WRITER	Steve Halliday, PhD
INTERNAL PEER REVIEWERS	Donald L. Jernigan, PhD
	Michael Cacciatore, MD
EXTERNAL PEER REVIEWERS	Lewis Sorley, PhD
	Stephen S. Favaloro
COPY EDITOR	Pam Nordberg
PROMOTION	Caryn McCleskey
PRODUCTION	Lillian Boyd
PHOTOGRAPHY	Spencer Freeman
COVER DESIGN	Kirk DouPonce

For special orders, events, or other information, please contact:
AdventHealthPress.com | 407-200-8224

AdventHealth Press is a wholly owned entity of AdventHealth.
Library of Congress Control Number: 2015957677
Printed in the United States of America.
PR 14 13 12 11 10 9 8 7 6 5 4 3
ISBN 978-0-7953480-8-2 (Print)
ISBN 978-0-9996983-8-9 (EBook)

For other life-changing resources please visit:
AdventHealthPress.com
CREATIONLife.com

Dedicated to those on the front line of healthcare:
— The doctors, nurses, clinicians, administrators —
Who are my new "battle buddies" in this, my second career.
They are in every way of the same selfless ilk
Of the heroes I previously served alongside.

CONTENTS

FOREWORD

Hospitals and clinics worldwide deserve to be led by top-notch ethical leaders—and Mark Hertling knows a great deal about ethical leadership. A graduate of the United States Military Academy at West Point with almost four decades of service in the U.S. Army, Mark has taken his leadership education, experiences, and insights and provided healthcare professionals with a brilliant, easy-to-understand book on leadership in healthcare.

The leadership lessons and tips in *Growing Physician Leaders*, when applied by physicians, hospitals, and healthcare systems, will improve healthcare and patient care across America. Timing is everything, and this terrific read is just what current and future leaders in healthcare need to help them develop and lead themselves, their patients, their staffs, and their teams (in clinics, operating rooms, staff meetings, or any other part of the healthcare system).

Auspiciously for an author of a book on physician leadership, Mark began his military career as a patient. Shortly after graduating from West Point, as a young second lieutenant in Germany, Mark underwent emergency orthopedic surgery for a double compound fracture that almost cost him his leg. His surgeon was John Feagin, the namesake, benefactor, and inspiration for our leadership program for medical students and residents at Duke University. Mark and John both went on to distinguished military and medical careers where they were recognized as two of the most caring, competent, knowledgeable, selfless, and enthusiastic leaders our country has been honored to have. Now, over 40 years after their initial meeting as patient and surgeon, both are committed to teaching leadership skills for the complex challenges facing healthcare—John Feagin through his commitment to the Feagin Leadership Program, and Mark through this book and his commitment to the challenging task of teaching leadership skills to physicians in the AdventHealth system. Mark's leadership course at AdventHealth and this book are "just what the doctor ordered."

In *Growing Physician Leaders*, Mark shares many of the leadership lessons he learned, taught, and practiced during his years in the U.S. Army. Ethical leadership is the heart and soul of our nation's military and it is in the DNA of every soldier, sailor, airman, Coast Guardsman, and marine. Our military is recognized worldwide for its ethical leadership and the military is one of the most, if not the most, trusted institutions in America. As such, it makes perfect sense to take the best leadership practices from the military and apply them in a healthcare context. Mark Hertling has done just that.

For some it may seem strange to have a non-healthcare professional writing and teaching about leadership in the healthcare field—especially a military leader such as Mark. However, as we have found in teaching leadership skills in the Feagin Leadership Program, there are many competencies that overlap between the military and medicine. In fact, the five core competencies in the research-derived Duke Healthcare Leadership Model—emotional intelligence, teamwork, selfless service, critical thinking, and integrity—are competencies that are also taught and emphasized in the military, as Mark so clearly describes.

The timing and need for leadership development both in healthcare and academic medicine are clear. The gap in leadership development in medicine is well known and is only now starting to be intentionally addressed. Healthcare professionals need leadership skills to improve care for patients and patient populations, to improve access to healthcare for all demographics, and to reduce cost while addressing these requirements.

One of the many strengths of *Growing Physician Leaders* is that it has leadership lessons for the beginner, novice, intermediate, and experienced leader. The lessons run the spectrum from the one-on-one relationship level to the strategic and visionary levels of leadership. Additionally, Mark's use of stories is a powerful and effective technique for readers to understand, feel, and better internalize the many competencies and traits that effective ethical leaders should practice.

Congratulations and kudos to Mark for sharing his lifelong leadership lessons with us in this wonderful book. We are confident you will benefit greatly on your own leadership development journey from the help of *Growing Physician Leaders*.

JOE DOTY, PHD
DEAN TAYLOR, MD
JOHN FEAGIN, MD
Feagin Leadership Program
Duke University

PREFACE

From the Battlefield to the Medical Field

After an extremely satisfying four-decade career in the US Army, I hung up my uniform and put away my combat boots and wondered what I ought to do next. My wife and I knew that retirement from the army would bring new adventures, but I felt anxious. Would we find the "family," the mission, the values, the energy, and the passion in the private sector that would equal what we had experienced for so many years in the military?

While many of my peers opt for second careers in the defense industry or as independent consultants, I didn't want to walk either of those paths. I wanted to make a different kind of contribution, although I didn't know quite where, what, or how.

Through a series of coincidences, I met a group of dedicated and impressive professionals from AdventHealth, one of the largest admitting hospitals in America (and the lead facility in the largest Protestant healthcare group in the nation). They and their colleagues face a cluster of daunting challenges and, they believed, a retired general from a different vocational background might be able to help them overcome those challenges.

To make a long story short, I enlisted.

Soon after I signed on, the chief operating officer and chief medical officer began a conversation with me about the topic of leadership. Both men had for a long time wanted to find ways to help doctors become better leaders so they could more effectively contribute to the goals and culture of the organization, yet both admitted they hadn't found the right approach or the right program. They had tried sending physicians to a variety of courses at other organizations. That tactic didn't work. They had contracted for consultants to work as coaches with specific physicians currently in leadership roles. But that approach didn't get them the results they needed, either.

How could they infuse the hospital with physicians who had great medical skills, they wondered, *and* who understood and endorsed the vision, the mission, and the values of their organization? They wanted team-oriented leaders willing to tackle the myriad challenges of contemporary healthcare. I'd told them that for decades, in both formal and informal settings, I had helped young army officers grow in their understanding and exercise of leadership.

"Do you think you could design a program for us to help doctors grow professionally and personally as leaders?" they asked. Now, in many ways, leadership is leadership, whether in the military or in healthcare. So after assessing the new challenge, I told them I thought I could.

We set out to design and execute a Physician Leader Course. After leading several groups of doctors, nurses, and administrators through the class, we have already seen some remarkably positive cultural and organizational shifts take place because of what these motivated healthcare workers have learned and applied. Our chief medical officer has called the course we designed "catastrophically successful," as it has contributed to transformational change in course participants and among those who have observed their passionate and informed contribution.

We have seen our graduates—doctors, nurses, and administrators—come to a deeper understanding of what true leadership entails, while also demonstrating a desire to apply those insights in ways that make a crucial, helpful difference. Because of the skills our participants have learned, they are now volunteering for and getting asked to lead in various positions and in varied contexts. We also are now tracking data that shows how recent class graduates and current class participants are actively seeking leadership positions within our organization and within the larger world of healthcare.

This book is based largely on the core content developed for our Physician Leadership Course. It lays out what I believe any leader must know and apply, whether that leader directs troops on a battlefield or guides specialized teams in a hospital. AdventHealth has now enthusiastically taken on the mission of growing effective leaders and key contributors for healthcare across the country.

We are in the early stages of some formal research to determine reportable effects of the leadership course on measurable performance indicators, such as patient experience feedback, HCAHP (Hospital Consumer Assessment of Healthcare Providers and Systems) scores, and treatment effectiveness. Already we're getting reports of significant changes in the way physicians engage with their patients and the patients' families, their colleagues, and with administrators in the patient's room, in an operating suite, or on teams focused on solving the critical challenges facing healthcare.

This book represents my attempt to take my experience in growing leaders in the army and adapting those insights for the specialized world of healthcare. I believe the results we've already seen at AdventHealth will continue to multiply throughout our system, and I hope what we have learned will also inspire other hospitals and healthcare organizations throughout the nation to follow a similar track. We want to help talented physicians reach their top potential as doctors and become the excellent healthcare leaders they have the capacity to become. Equally as important, perhaps, we want to help them experience the thrill of effectively leading others in a war we can't afford to lose.

MARK HERTLING
Lieutenant General, US Army (Ret.)
Senior Vice President, AdventHealth

INTRODUCTION

What to Know before You Begin

America needs a nationwide reveille to find ways to improve its healthcare system—and doctors must lead the charge.

It didn't take me long to get that message once I retired from the US Army and began a second career in the American healthcare industry. I heard it from my new colleagues. I observed it in my new setting. And whenever I picked up a medical journal or professional article, I seemed to find at least one article proclaiming how "physicians must lead!"

But while doctors certainly know how to care for their patients, and while a growing nationwide chorus of voices is pleading for physicians to become better leaders, we have a huge problem to overcome. From my perspective as a military veteran and a relative newbie to healthcare, *I see little opportunity for physicians to learn how to lead.*

It's not that physicians don't want to lead. They do.

It's not that administrators don't need them to lead. They do.

The problem is that medical schools don't teach leadership skills and that most healthcare organizations lack viable training opportunities to help their physicians become effective leaders. Although many doctors have innate leadership skills and seek ways to improve them, I hear continually from frustrated physicians and administrators who tell me they can't find a good class or training program that will help them further develop as leaders and more effectively take on the reins of leadership. They protest that while they have no difficulty finding schools of management or business administration that offer instruction on processes, systems, negotiation, communication skills, and the like, they've looked in vain for potent, organized approaches that teach and train the basic principles of leadership.

As someone who has spent a career continuously improving my leadership skills, or training others to improve their leadership abilities, I find all of this intriguing. And it represents a key difference between how the medical profession and how the military profession prepare their respective leaders.

The military formally educates and trains soldiers in the art of leadership using a progressive, organized, and formalized three-tiered approach that involves instruction, operational experience, and self-learning. Not so the healthcare profession. Other than episodic lectures and courses or occasional seminars on specific management skills and processes, healthcare typically does not engage in systematic, ongoing, designed episodes of leadership education and training. Even many of the leadership initiatives I have seen in healthcare appear more geared toward management techniques than leadership development. But leadership is different from management, and while the two often intersect, the basics of leadership must be presented differently.

How Would the Army Deal with This?

Dr. Dave Moorhead, the chief medical officer at AdventHealth and a man of strong principles, has a thousand ideas about how to make healthcare better. He also has a clear vision that healthcare executives must do a better job of training physicians in leadership skills.

Dave took me under his wing after I arrived at AdventHealth Orlando. He expressed a fascination with my career as a soldier and wanted to learn more about it, perhaps because he recognized that good organizations proactively look outside their own cultures for new ways to address old problems. He also felt thankful that his boss and mine, the chief operating officer of AdventHealth Orlando, Brian Paradis, had recruited and hired a retired general to provide a different cultural approach to healthcare issues. Dave also observed, rightly, that I seemed equally fascinated with his successful career as a doctor and teacher, and he felt happy to become my mentor as I learned the intricacies of healthcare.

AdventHealth Orlando had hired me to develop a new initiative centered on global partnering, to help find ways to work with other countries as a means of sharing ideas about population health. While I busied myself with that program, Dave frequently dropped in to discuss leadership issues. He would tell me about a tough challenge facing a team on one of our campuses, or confide about a disciplinary matter in which the medical staff struggled to uphold the organization's standards, or describe a difficult relationship with someone at another healthcare organization, made worse by a lack of communication skills. He would always ask, "How would you deal with this kind of problem in the army?"

After one pleasant but lengthy discussion about the differences in leadership training between healthcare and the military, Dave made a startling admission that truly shocked me. "You've really helped me to understand why leadership issues are such a challenge in the medical profession," he said carefully. "In medicine, we haven't grown our physicians to be leaders. In fact, we take pride in a system that actually tends to beat out of our doctors any ability they might have as a leader. We do this from the time they enter med school, through their residency, and into their practices. We do it through excessive demands, messages on how much workload and patient throughput they should have, competition for specialty and subspecialty selection—all without any formal approach to leadership training. And then we scratch our heads and say we don't understand why physicians can't lead our healthcare organizations."

The military model, by contrast, follows a simple progression: Learn the basics in the schoolhouse; apply those basics in operational assignments; continuously grow every day through self-study and self-assessment. Then, turn up the rheostat and add more complexity and an ever-increasing array of challenges in successive learning environments. Wash-rinse-repeat.

The way leaders get chosen also differs significantly in the two professions. In the healthcare industry, Dave told me, physicians often get chosen or hired for top positions based almost entirely on their reputation for excellent medical skill, or on the length and impressiveness of their published work, or on which groups they've talked to as outlined in their CVs. Rarely do they get recruited for how they analyze human dynamics, engage with and inform patients, form teams, build consensus, communicate vision, and influence others to achieve the organization's stated goals.

By contrast, the military recognizes that leading organizations is a learned "art." While both soldiers and doctors must possess technical skills and understand "science," the profession of arms places a significant amount of emphasis on *growing* military leaders.

As Dave pondered these substantial differences, in time he asked me directly: "Could we apply this model to physicians in order to help them become better leaders, and in that way address more critical issues in healthcare?" I thought we could; and so we began developing a Physician Leadership Development (PLD) course, which provided the core content for this book.

Getting Started

With the help of Lee Johnson, who had worked with physicians her entire career, and a newly hired military colleague, Colonel [retired] Jay Voorhees, who had led aviation units in both the conventional and Special Operations forces, and using the Army Leadership Manual as a guide, we developed a course for our first class of thirty-five physicians, ten clinicians, and five hospital administrators.

The seminar included a mix of various physician specialties (surgeons, primary care physicians, radiologists, internists, cardiovascular specialists, anesthesiologists, etc.) that evenly represented all of our campuses. A small group of nurses, clinicians, and hospital administrators joined them.

The key lessons from that course led to the key questions in this book:

- *What is leadership, and why must physicians become better leaders?*

- *How does developing a stronger sense of professionalism empower leadership?*

- *What attributes and competencies do all true leaders share?*

- *How do leaders build effective teams?*

- *How can physicians better lead their organizations?*

- *What kind of healthcare leaders will transform healthcare?*

As we explore these critical issues in *Growing Physician Leaders*, I'll frequently return to the real-world results we've already seen at

AdventHealth Orlando as our doctors and healthcare professionals have put into practice what they learned in the PLD course. We'll also hear directly from them and from some of their coworkers, describing how their new leadership skills have enabled them to achieve breakthroughs and enjoy success in problematic areas that once caused them significant distress.

While I didn't write this book to provide a comprehensive analysis of the many leadership challenges facing healthcare—far from it—I did tackle the project to demonstrate two simple but crucial truths. First, I wanted to show how applying a few basic leadership tenets in a healthcare environment can radically change those environments for the better. And second, I wanted to show how *any* physician or healthcare professional can learn to become a more effective leader, resulting in greater standards of achievement and higher levels of satisfaction... for everyone involved.

What's With the War Stories?

Finally, if you've looked at the Table of Contents, you've seen a number of "War Stories" listed. Why would I include war stories from my military career in a book addressed to physicians and other healthcare professionals?

As a way to keep the attention of young soldiers, many military leaders tell "war stories" to influence, inspire, and encourage their troops. Telling tales of men, myths, legends, tense situations, and those who went before always gets a warm welcome in training or combat environments. When those hearing the stories face some frightening situation for the first time, believe me, they want to know that others have successfully confronted similar challenges!

War stories also can be used to introduce an idea, break the tension, perhaps provide some laughs, or emphasize an important teaching point. That's why they always start with the phrase, "So there we were..." The phrase warns the listener, "Listen up, because a war story is about to begin!"

Most commanders use war stories throughout their military careers, in both formal and informal situations. Tim O'Brien, in his excellent fictional work about Vietnam titled *The Things They Carried*, suggests that in war stories nothing is absolutely true, because often it's difficult to separate what actually happened from what seemed to happen. While I've never condoned lying, telling a war story allows for "bending facts," so long as it has a moral or a key objective (or a surprise punch line). Good storytellers conjure up believable tales of heroism, selfless service, courage, and perseverance in the midst of overwhelming circumstances, so that soldiers will believe they also can accomplish the impossible.

And then those emboldened soldiers go out and accomplish exactly that.

Every war story has myriad truths, morals, and emotions, if we can discover and meditate on them. Stories drive understanding. A good anecdote can powerfully illustrate an important principle and can even inspire and influence others to learn and change the direction of their lives.

As a professional soldier who has either observed or participated in the kind of stressful situations that easily work as real-life war stories, it's natural for me to use such stories whenever I try to explain leadership, regardless of the setting. Throughout this book, then, I will tell a few selected war stories to highlight the leadership principles I'm about to discuss. I've learned the tactic works well with physicians, perhaps because war stories closely resemble the "cases" doctors often relate when trying to establish immediate professional respect and rapport with new colleagues or teams. Their interactions often begin with something like, "Let me tell you about a case I had awhile ago"—the medical-speak equivalent of, "So there we were."

As we begin, be on the lookout for the venerable opening phrase, "So there we were…" I tell these stories not just to relive old times, but to hammer home some crucial principle. And if you find yourself entertained along the way, then so much the better.

Time to "Ruck Up"

I end this introduction with the claim that began it: training physicians in basic leadership skills is a key to improving our overall healthcare system. I hope the insights in this book might prove valuable to physicians and healthcare leaders, but I also hope my observations about how physicians might become better leaders will find a much broader audience than the solitary group addressed in the title. Perhaps policy makers, pharmaceutical chains, medical supply companies, politicians, and every patient, consumer, or observer of healthcare will find insight into how physician leaders can improve healthcare across the spectrum in the United States.

But I also would like to add a promise, one I know to be true: *Leadership can be learned, regardless of the person, the venue, the profession, or the work environment.*

And now I'd like to show you how.

CHAPTER 1

Why Physicians Need to Lead

M any people are under the impression that leaders are born, not made.

It's not completely true.

For decades, I watched as young soldiers learned the intricacies of leadership and then went out and led others effectively in all sorts of challenging environments. While one person might have more natural gifts as a leader, the fact is that really good leaders are made, not born.

And that includes physicians.

But why should physicians *want* to become better leaders? Why add one more responsibility on top of all the others they already possess? How can learning the art of leadership help them, their patients, and their organizations to thrive?

The Challenge of the Triple Aim

Many doctors may feel tempted to think, *Why should I spend a lot of time interacting with a patient, a patient's family, or other members of a healthcare team, when I could be putting in extra effort honing my skills and techniques? Shouldn't everyone simply understand that the important things are my board certification, my title, the knowledge I've amassed from so much training, my appointed position in a practice or in this hospital, and my curriculum vitae?* Armed with such a mindset, many doctors see leadership skills as nice to have but secondary to their practice of medicine.

And in fact, from the beginning of their training, physicians are taught to focus so strongly on the *science* of their profession—how to fix problems and make people better—that they often don't pay as much attention to the *art* of interpersonal relationships. As someone who has been tasked with leading tens of thousands of men and women through life and death situations, however, I know that cultivating such relationships and building trust with others is the very essence of leadership. And during a time when healthcare faces a host of growing challenges, it is an absolute requirement.

Physicians, hospitals, and a variety of healthcare organizations rightfully worry about how we as a nation will address the elements of what is commonly known as the **Triple Aim**:

1. Increase access to healthcare for all demographics.
2. Reduce costs associated with medical expenses.
3. Improve care for patients and populations.

While the daunting challenges connected with the Triple Aim are worth a book in themselves, let me sketch out two of the biggest issues related to physicians and leadership.

First is the distance of physicians from leadership (i.e., policy-making) roles. In this country we have, and will continue to have, negative trend lines linked to deteriorating health conditions, such as obesity, diabetes, complex care issues for the aged, behavioral health concerns, and a plethora of other issues related to acute care.[1] While doctors are on the front line of this battle defending against disease and finding ways to improve care and access, physicians often find themselves disconnected from the policies and procedures that help accomplish the Triple Aim. Why this disconnect? Often, physicians don't get included—they don't even get a seat at the table—because those in charge don't see them as leaders.

Second is the issue of finances. The financial challenges our nation faces in healthcare resemble, in many ways, the difficulties we face in the arena of defense spending. While both are linked to national security and a concern for our future economic well-being, I suspect most Americans believe the Department of Defense far outpaces healthcare on spending, as a percentage of gross domestic product (GDP). But in fact, the percent of our GDP spent on healthcare dwarfs the amount spent on national defense. According to the World Health Organization, total healthcare spending in the US was 17.9 percent of GDP in 2011, the highest in the world.[2] The Health and Human Services Department expects that the health share of GDP will continue its historical upward trend, reaching 19.5 percent of GDP by 2017.[2] In effect, the percentage of our GDP linked to various aspects of healthcare is almost *five times* what our nation spends on defense, which continuously and historically hovers right around 4 percent.[3]

Since physicians know in detail many of the critical issues related to our nation's health, they are the ones best positioned to contribute to providing workable solutions to address and solve these challenges— *if* they learn to effectively lead. Today, however, physicians are mostly removed from leadership roles. While they provide excellent care to patients in treatment facilities and operating suites, they often do not provide needed input in regard to strategic vision and organizational direction. Most hospitals in the US have nonphysician managers as their chief executive officers, with one report claiming that physicians led only 235 of 6,500 hospitals in the nation.[4]

Physicians *must* play a more significant role in the tactical and strategic running of our healthcare institutions. This will occur, to everyone's benefit, as our doctors gain the leadership skills they need to better relate to one another and to other healthcare professionals and administrators. Our physicians rightly want a seat at the table, but in order to gain that seat, they must first learn the required "table manners" associated with leading others, leading teams, and building effective and efficient organizations.

A Lesson from Sun Tzu

One of history's great military theorists is the Chinese general and philosopher Sun Tzu. His insights are preserved in the great work *The Art of War*, which somehow found popularity in corporate America in the 1980s. After his name got mentioned in several popular films, business executives began citing his work, often taking his quotations out of context and applying his philosophy to competition strategies, market approaches, and methods of building organizations ready for any challenge. Most leaders in the private sector these days are aware of the classic work, and even of Sun Tzu's words, but often don't adequately apply the philosophy.

The military takes Sun Tzu's words and puts them into action, especially one of his primary dicta, employed at all of its training centers: "Know the enemy, know the terrain, and know yourself; in a thousand battles you will never be defeated." In the army, we took a systematic approach to addressing each of those critical issues to help us prepare for victory.

Shortly after I arrived at AdventHealth Orlando, I was asked to take a look around the organization and give my assessment of what the hospital needed to do to grow physician leaders. I had begun to learn something of the national challenges doctors face in becoming better leaders, but my new employer wanted to get a retired general's perspective on the state of its own physician leaders. I therefore agreed to observe the practices, the clinics, the physician lounges, and the healthcare teams as they executed their work on the eight campuses of AdventHealth Orlando, and then present an analysis as to what we could do that seemed both helpful and possible. In Sun Tzu's parlance, I wanted to get a good idea of *ourselves* (how the physicians led), the *terrain* (the hospital and healthcare environment), and the *enemy* (what was preventing doctors from becoming better leaders). How did we function as leaders, and how did we view ourselves as leaders, based on the environment? Any healthcare organization considering a leadership assessment could greatly benefit from such an approach.

I quickly found that each of the eight campuses of AdventHealth Orlando has its own personality, designed to serve unique and varied patient demographics and run by very different administrators. Some facilities have large medical staffs, others have much smaller ones; some hospital administrators are hands-on and centralized, others have a more decentralized approach.

The system has what some term a "hybrid medical staff," with contract physicians, contributing physician groups, hospitalists, and private practice physicians. While some physicians practice primarily at or near one of our campuses, others travel between hospitals. The system has many superb "permanent" teams, some ad hoc teams, and a few teams that many would call dysfunctional. After a three-week assessment, I determined several things.

First, AdventHealth is a values-based, learning and growing organization. Its stated mission to "extend the healing ministry of Christ" is clear and well understood. Its vision—becoming a world-class organization that continuously addresses healthcare's Triple Aim of increased access, reduced cost, and better care—appears to contribute to continued improvement and innovation. I observed an excellent connection with the community and noted high patient engagement evaluations. I saw many talented and dedicated physicians, and I sensed a strong desire for constant adaptation in caring for our patients and their families.

On the other hand, while I observed extremely well-skilled and highly competent doctors, I didn't see enough of them leading. On too many occasions, I watched them fail to communicate effectively with team members, with patients, and with patient families. Many displayed a distrust of the executive staff, and the majority appeared to have little idea how to build strong teams. I observed a few examples of toxic leadership behavior and heard a few stories from nurses about doctors throwing tantrums in the operating room or of unprofessional dialogue with workers and inappropriate behavior when asked to perform coordinating tasks.

(I later learned that our conduct review boards often handled cases like these. And I learned that most hospitals struggle with the same issues.)

In speaking directly to a variety of healthcare professionals, including doctors, clinicians, and administrators, I discovered that most used but could not accurately define the key terms of management (systems and control processes) and leadership (methods of engaging people to voluntarily work together to achieve organizational goals). In fact, I found no clear understanding or definition of leadership or of how good leadership could contribute to organizational excellence.

My research and analysis led me to conclude that although the hospital wanted true leadership training specifically for physicians, such training did not seem to exist. While nearly everyone I spoke to had expressed a desire for effective training to help physicians become better leaders, no one seemed to know where to find it.

Additionally, I discovered that, in many cases, physicians were not considered a part of the official healthcare team, which meant they often got overlooked for management and leadership training courses and opportunities. In other words, the hospital not only lacked good training opportunities, but our physicians often expressed frustration at getting left out of the formal professional development programs offered to clinicians and administrators (usually through the human resources program). It's tough to ask physicians to take on more leadership roles when they have few processes, systems, or training opportunities to prepare them for leading.

Finally, I discovered that while the hospital sometimes sent physicians to various seminars described as leadership courses, whether at universities or outside groups, these classes did not happen in systematic ways, did not provide a program that understood our culture or was applied directly to our situation, and did not appear to have a lasting effect on the organization.

As I wrapped up my assessment, I couldn't help but note that the military uses a very different model to choose and equip its own leaders. Officers and noncommissioned officers (the "sergeants") receive ongoing education on leadership principles and theory, along with increasingly technical skills training associated with their specific job requirements. From the beginning, a young second lieutenant or sergeant learns the basics of leadership attributes, competencies, styles, and techniques. While added rank and increasingly complex assignments might bring more difficult leadership challenges, the leadership "basics" remain unchanged, even as they get applied in different scenarios.

The military education system, with its focus on leadership fundamentals applied at each level, allows individuals to grow professionally and personally in their leadership abilities. After graduating from these various courses, military leaders are required to engage with others, build teams, develop their people, and succeed with their particular organization in each successive operational assignment. When soldiers aren't learning leadership in schools or practicing the art of leadership in their organizations, they are expected to participate in continuous self-study and self-assessment.

As I pondered the differences in leadership training between what I'd experienced in the military and what I'd seen in healthcare, I realized my new challenge required me to sharpen exactly what I meant by "leadership." In the army, we lived and breathed its principles every day; but in my new environment, how could I hope to improve the general level of leadership of our organization if many of my students didn't even share a clear concept of what it was and what it involved? And so I began to refine how to describe "the ideal leader."

What Does the "Ideal Leader" Look Like?

A few years ago, I participated in a conference at West Point designed to gain consensus on the elements of leadership, in preparation for re-publishing our service's leadership manual (known as *Army Doctrine Reference Publication*, or ADRP 6-22).[5] Some of us more senior folks kiddingly called this conference a SEE, or Significant Emotional Event. We knew what we would be discussing and how it applied, but the event was necessary to start gaining consensus and enforcing our cultural understanding of leadership.

Over the course of a few days, and in deep discussion of the profession of arms and the leadership requirements of that profession, many attendees refined their view of the ideal leader. After the conference, I could succinctly and accurately understand and define the term "leadership" as used in the army.

A practical reason lay behind this conference. After almost ten years of war in Iraq and Afghanistan, our chief of staff, the top general in the army, felt troubled by the conduct of some of our officers and soldiers. A few acts of indiscipline and misconduct in the ranks had become public knowledge, along with a few similar incidents among our senior leaders. The Abu Ghraib scandal and a few embarrassing sexual dalliances involving senior leaders appeared to be anomalies; but as an organization, we needed to ensure that we reframed the fundamentals of appropriate army behavior and values.

The chief wanted his senior leaders to review the elements of the profession of arms and then come to a consensus on the role army leaders play in ensuring that the organization meets its own standards, serves our soldiers, and serves our nation. A variety of army senior leaders, professors of military ethics and leadership, and retired general officers (those we call "gray beards" due to their knowledge and reflections) participated in this unique event.

Like all good soldiers, I always kept a green notebook nearby, which

I had with me during this conference. In the army, these ubiquitous notebooks contain our notes on assigned tasks, missions, and information from critical meetings that need to get passed along to subordinates. "A short pencil is always better than a longer memory," a sergeant once told me as a young lieutenant.

These notebooks always have a section that most use to jot down provocative thoughts. I enjoy periodically reviewing my old notes, because I usually come across something interesting. So before I began designing the Physician Leadership Development (PLD) course for our physician leaders, I thought it might be a good idea to dust off this particular notebook and review what I had learned at this conference.

As soon as I opened it, I saw one especially striking entry. It suggested that one needed to define the ideal before trying to define the attributes and characteristics of leadership. I read the following:

> An ideal leader has a strong intellect, a physical presence, a continuously developing professional competence, a refined moral character, and he or she must realize they are always serving as an example to others. A leader must be willing to act decisively, exhibit courage and candor when required, and do all of this in the best interest of the organization. Leaders have the primary requirement to build trust and confidence, because the leader can then use that trust to get things done. If the leader does all these things, he or she will successfully care for his or her soldiers, build strong teams, and accomplish any task, no matter how difficult.

My notes almost perfectly reflected the text that found its way into the manual a year later. That description clearly defined what the ideal army leader strives to be, to know, and to do throughout a military career.

When I read my notes again several years after I wrote down that definition, I had a strong reaction. *Wow*, I thought, *this applies perfectly in defining the ideal physician leader, someone who selflessly and humbly serves patients and the healthcare organization.* It struck me that physicians also need to understand and strive to meet the ideals of *being, knowing,* and *doing.*

A Working Definition of Leadership

While having a description of an ideal leader can provide something like a beacon, giving light in foggy places, a concise working definition of the word "leadership" can be even more useful, especially in contexts where no such definition has widely existed. I already had seen that many of my colleagues at AdventHealth intermingled the terms "leadership" and "management," so I knew early on we needed to eliminate some confusion.

Most business schools rely on some variant of Webster's definition of management when teaching systems and processes. Webster's defines management as "the organization and coordination of the activities of a business in order to achieve defined objectives." While one might make the argument that human interaction is inherent in any "coordination of activities," management seems to be more about systems and processes than about trust and influence, both of which fall into the realm of leadership. Management teaches that if one puts things in proper sequence and applies precise rules and boundaries, then one can achieve organizational goals.

To me, this seems to imply that management is about *what you do.* A good manager might analyze how to improve a cost-benefit ratio for insurance coverage, or find ways to reduce the wait time in an emergency room, or find more efficient methods of patient payment models, or determine the effectiveness of a human resource policy. If he or she does all these things, then the organization likely will achieve some increased level of success.

But long ago, after four decades in the military, I concluded that leadership is far more important because it is about *who we are*. It is about the leader and it is about those being led. It is also about the interaction between the two.

Someone who desires to be a leader must first know himself or herself. True leaders must look deep inside to see who they are. They must refine what they believe in order to understand how they interact. Then, the aspiring leader must learn how to listen, so he or she can determine what motivates an individual, a team, or an organization.

The individual who wants to be a leader must also first understand and then learn to apply a variety of influence techniques—the right technique at the right time in the right place—in order to give purpose and direction to one person or to a group of people. The leader must know how to communicate vision, goals, and objectives on a grand scale to a large organization, but he or she must also know the fine art of understanding and communicating with every individual member of the team.

How do you get all of *that* into a succinct definition that can be discussed and debated and applied over a long period of time by a group of highly accomplished healthcare professionals? It's a challenge! I therefore looked in the army's leadership manual once again and slightly edited its definition to provide a starting point:

> Leadership is the art of understanding motivations, influencing people and teams, and communicating purpose and direction to accomplish stated goals while improving the organization.

That's about as good a working definition as I can devise. Like all working definitions, it can be edited and adjusted and applied to various circumstances and scenarios involving different individuals and teams. Let's briefly break down this version to see how it works.

Motivation is intrinsic by nature. I personally don't believe in extrinsic motivation, but I do believe a leader can *influence* others using a variety of techniques. *Purpose* (some call it *vision*) gives the individual or the team a reason to seek a desired outcome. The way the leader *communicates*, using a variety of oral and written methods in a variety of theatrical or nontheatrical ways, is critical to success. *Accomplishing stated goals* and *improving the organization* is the raison d'être for leadership.

I intentionally describe leadership as an "art." I've learned that one can have a perfectly "scientific" understanding of leadership, based on a thousand peer-reviewed studies, but unless one masters the art of interacting with human beings, those leadership "facts" will do little good. And physician leaders have to interact with a lot of individuals! They must deal daily with patients, patients' families, fellow healthcare team members in the clinical and administrative areas, and executives in the large organization, to name just a few.

No single approach or easy solution exists to solving the challenges and issues associated with the wide variety of human interaction. But a simple leadership model that focuses on the art of leadership—keeping in mind the constantly changing dynamics of motivation, methods of influence, means of communication, and evaluation of organizational accomplishment—can help physician leaders to achieve a level of success in their organizations that frankly astounds them, once they apply it.

Key Elements of Our Leadership Model

A mentor once told me that one of the key principles of strategic communication is the ability to describe difficult concepts in an uncomplicated way. So how do you make leadership simple?

As I reflected on the essence of leadership, I landed on several things that *all* leaders, regardless of their profession or line of work, need to understand:

Good leaders know themselves; they are conscious of who they are and what they stand for. They know the specific values they hold. All leaders come to realize that the crucial ingredient of leadership is finding multiple ways to build trust.

Leaders understand the fundamental, trust-based nature of leadership. Good leaders define leadership for themselves and can apply that definition to interactions with individuals, with their teams, and within their organization. Leaders know they must possess specific attributes and competencies and realize they must get better at surmounting their deficiencies. Leaders determine their personal values and know how those values contribute to decision making throughout the leadership journey. And leaders know that all of these factors working together contribute to generating trust—and they recognize trust as the basic component of leadership. Therefore, the first step to growing leaders is helping them to better see themselves.

Good leaders understand dyadic interaction and how leading teams, even in a large organization, begins with leading one person at a time.

Leadership is hard! It also requires a great deal of work. While the concepts in this book might assist individuals in learning how to formally and informally lead other individuals, teams, and even large organizations, any leader who wants to succeed in any organization, regardless of its size, needs to first learn how to lead just one other person. That one other person might be a patient or someone in a patient's family, a part of the leader's team, or a peer or colleague. Or it could be the leader's boss, which requires the leader to learn how to "lead up" (a term popularized by Michael Useem in his book of the same title).

The "leading up" principle is particularly important to physician leaders and will become increasingly important as physicians begin to make larger contributions to a profession that often has not placed trained leaders in crucial roles. Leading up is required when physicians informally engage with hospital administrators or nonphysician healthcare professionals.

Applying principles of one-on-one leadership to larger groups eventually will contribute to physicians having an even more profound effect than they already do in influencing the actions of their patients. It also will play a key role in shaping the attitudes and decisions of those in charge of healthcare organizations. To achieve such a profound effect, the physician leader must develop appropriate skills that will help him or her gain greater empathy, while also acquiring greater insight as to how to communicate in such a way that those being led will see a particular problem from a different perspective. By understanding the motivations of a patient, a team, or a boss, and by using a variety of influence techniques, all sides (and especially the patient!) will win.

Dyadic (or "one-on-one") leadership must be mastered before any leader attempts to extend his or her leadership abilities to address bigger challenges or larger organizations.

Good leaders understand how to build and lead teams in various situations.

Knowing how to define leadership, understanding what motivates those being led, and using various influence techniques all vary depending on the size and nature of the group, the individual's motivations, how the leader uses various influence methods, and the type of group being led. A physician might feel comfortable leading a small team with whom he or she works daily. In the operating room, a surgeon tends to rely heavily on a relatively small surgical nursing staff, highly trained technicians, and an experienced anesthesiologist. But to address larger healthcare issues, an approach that works well with a well-oiled team may not work at all with a large group in a boardroom, whose members all possess varying (and not always evident) motivations.

Physician leaders must learn to broaden their approach. They must consider the motivations of a variety of people largely unknown to them, apply relevant influence techniques, assess group cohesion, and use approaches appropriate to the specific assignment, whether large groups or small groups, hospital administrators or clinicians, government officials or various other professionals.

Good leaders are good team players.

To succeed, good leaders realize that no matter where they land in an organization, they always depend on others, just as others depend on them. Leadership is a team sport, which means that everyone wins together or loses together. No one can do anything significant without the help of others—and true leaders have a commitment to contributing to the success of all.

In the healthcare arena, physicians live at the center of the universe because they connect with the patient. But others also inhabit that universe: hospital executives and government administrators, lawyers, human resource champions, insurers, transporters, clinicians, researchers, and a host of others. All of them are members of the same team, and all of them ultimately serve the patient and contribute to healthcare.

Physician leaders need to learn what the hospital does for them and how they can best contribute to their healthcare organizations. Since physicians can't win if their organizations lose, they must develop a stronger and bigger sense of team.

We'll look at all of these things in *Growing Physician Leaders*. Along the way, I'll also mention a few of the key elements in our Physician Leadership Development course that helped participants grasp and master these lessons. My goal throughout is to provide you with enough to get you started down the path of becoming a truly effective physician leader.

The Far Reach of Physician Leadership

The leadership principles in this book are not abstract concepts, untried in a medical setting. In fact, scores of physicians, nurses, and hospital administrators have now successfully completed the PLD course at AdventHealth Orlando, where they learned these principles and practiced these guidelines over a yearlong course. Graduates of the program are now finding practical applications for their leadership training in formal roles on our campuses and in their private practices, as well as on a variety of task forces that seek solutions to complex healthcare issues.

But perhaps the most encouraging concept for me is that I've found *physicians want to lead!* As one doctor told me after having a near-religious experience in the leadership class, "I've now realized, if you're not growing and learning new leadership skills every day, then something is wrong!"

When you learn to lead well and you apply sound leadership principles to every situation, then you can expect to be called repeatedly to lead, usually in increasingly complex circumstances. In the process, you'll learn more about leadership, no matter what role you may play or position of authority you may hold. And you *will* feel the satisfaction and have the thrill—I choose the word carefully—of providing the kind of effective leadership that gets things done.

Most leaders thrive on this unending cycle of learn, apply, and desire for more responsibility, and I hope it's something that causes your own heart to beat faster. Because, quite frankly, we need all the physician leaders we can find, grow, or attract.

WAR STORY

The *Wall Street Journal* Test

So there we were...

General Fred Franks had commanded the First Armored Division and then went on to command the famous US VII Corps during Operation Desert Storm. I had the honor of serving with him in both these organizations, first as his planner in the First Armored, then as a cavalry squadron operation officer in one of his units during Desert Storm. I saw General Franks as my mentor; he saw me as someone worthy of investment of his time and teaching.

When General Franks received his fourth star and took command of the army's Training and Doctrine Command (TRADOC)—the organization responsible for training, doctrine, leadership development, matériel design, and personnel requirements—he asked me to join him again. I held the rank of major and would serve as his speechwriter. He had a master's degree in English literature, and I had a master's in exercise physiology, so I knew I would learn much about writing speeches.

29

I didn't realize how much I would learn about leadership and profession-alism.

Beyond the crushing duties associated with charting the army's path in a variety of areas, General Franks made speeches, hosted award cere-monies, presented briefings, and presided over seminars to a wide variety of audiences several times a week. I would receive his guidance whenever his outer office received a speaking invitation, then conduct an audience analysis, work several drafts, and finally provide him with a product that he would often significantly edit. I found myself working three or four presentations at any given time, all at an unrelenting pace.

I worked hard, but for a great boss. General Franks always took the time to engage, coach, and counsel members of his team at every oppor-tunity. It was an honor to be allowed deep inside the strategic thought process of a senior army leader. He was assigned his own plane, so when he travelled around the country or the world, he normally asked me to join him as part of the traveling party. General Franks always made edits up to the last minute and would seek my help in thinking through those changes on the plane. But he always wanted a critique of how he delivered and how the audience had received his remarks. Even as one of the few four-star leaders at the peak of his career, he always looked for ways to improve.

One day, General Franks received an invitation to speak on a Friday afternoon to a class of more than one thousand young majors at Fort Leavenworth, Kansas. His secretary mentioned he felt doubly excited about this request, as his son-in-law was a member of the class. She told us he planned to spend the weekend with his daughter and his grandchildren after finishing the speech.

We had established a "battle drill" for preparing for these trips. My assistant would alert the pilots so they could start their flight planning, and then she began the travel and lodging arrangements while I began the audience analysis: the makeup of the college, the students' level of studies, what objectives the Leavenworth commandant wanted the general to cover. All of that linked to the message General Franks wanted to deliver. I soon had a topic outline that might help the boss refine his final guidance, which would in turn help me to start writing the first draft.

During our informal session the next morning, things went extremely well. He agreed with my outline and massaged it a bit with some specific details that came from his better understanding of the strategic landscape and the points he wanted to make. To conclude the session, as we always did, I covered the small administrative details of the trip—uniforms, when his aircraft would take off, when we would return, who would be in the traveling party, etc.

His ever-present smile faded. "Fellas," he said cordially, his smile returning as he realized there had been a disconnect in guidance, "the only two people going on this trip are my wife and me. Before all of you get your feelings hurt and think I'm snubbing my band of traveling brothers, understand there are all kinds of reasons, professional and personal, as to why none of you will accompany Denise [his wife] and me on this trip. And they are the same reasons we'll be taking a commercial plane and paying for the tickets out of our own pocket."

He had never done this before. Why buy a commercial plane ticket to travel to a military event, and why forego the support we provided to ensure an effective and efficient use of his time? His explanation gave us some insight into professionalism.

Leaders live on a glass pedestal in a glass house, he explained. Others are always watching to ensure your words match your actions and your actions line up with your values. As a leader, especially a senior leader with a lot of resources at his disposal to help him conduct the business of the army, he had to guard against anyone perceiving him as using his rank or his position for personal gain. What would others think if he were to use an army aircraft to fly to Kansas, and then those same people saw him playing in the park with his grandchildren on Saturday and Sunday?

"But boss," I protested, "they were the ones who invited you out there to speak! Why don't you take advantage of this opportunity? You spend so much time doing things on behalf of the army. Heck, if you were a CEO flying in your private jet, no one would think twice about you spending a few hours with your grandkids."

Again, he smiled that avuncular smile and took the time to mentor his stubborn protégé. "Yes, Mark," he said, "they invited me there to speak on Friday afternoon. But think this through. I address the class for an hour on Friday afternoon and I use that as an excuse to fly an army jet to Kansas on Friday and back on Sunday, while causing my aide and speechwriter—not to mention the pilot and copilot—to spend time away from their families, while I have a great time with my grandchildren? This is an army jet, not a corporate plane. The fuel for that jet is paid for by the people of the United States, as is the time of all those who would be pulled along with me. As a senior leader in the profession, I must be a steward of the organization."

Professionals must always consider the values of the profession, he continued, and we must hold ourselves accountable to the standards we set. Society must never lose trust in those charged with leading the profession of arms, because if that were to occur, the nation would surely crumble.

"It's the Wall Street Journal test, too," General Franks continued. "Imagine if some reporter got wind of me spending forty-eight hours with my grandkids. I could protest all I wanted about how I was invited to give a speech out there, but it just wouldn't fly when put under a microscope. And if that were published, it would tarnish the reputation of our profession. Besides, it isn't what 'right' looks like."

I'd never heard that phrase before, "What right looks like." Even though by that point I had been in the army for about a dozen years, I realized I needed to learn much more beyond shooting a tank, planning an operation, or any of the other skills of soldiering. We served in a profession critical to the health of the society; while others saw us as having tough standards, we held to those standards through some pretty tough self-policing. We had to live the values connected to the oath we took when joining the profession, and that required selfless service to our nation. As professionals, we had to remain continually aware of what right looked like.

CHAPTER 2

On Being Called a Professional

Believe it or not, soldiers and doctors have many things in common. As a career soldier, I got introduced to the importance of professional behavior the first time I put on a uniform. Even before I had a chance to study various works describing the elements of a profession or participate in discussions explaining the difference between a profession and a job, I was subjected to various elements of the profession of arms.

As a cadet at West Point, instructors and professors constantly used the word "professional" to describe those who performed according to the prescribed army standard in adherence to values, proper behavior, or performance of skills. Just as often, they used the term "unprofessional" as a sobriquet for anyone among us who suffered a lapse in judgment or displayed unsatisfactory behavior. The term became part of our lexicon, and not until I grew in rank and took on more extensive assignments did I have the opportunity to participate in more robust debate and discussion about the elements of a profession.

The more I studied the meaning of "profession" and the more I learned about what professionalism is all about, however, the more significant the concept became to me. Soon, I began to understand the key role that professionalism played in my career and the central importance of leadership in upholding all the elements of our profession, including the behavior expected of anyone in our profession.

Leaving One Profession for Another

When I left the military and began my new career in healthcare, I left one profession to join another. Yet early on, it seemed to me that many in healthcare who gladly took on the title of "professional" used that term without understanding the requirements associated with it. To me, being part of a profession and being called a professional meant more than merely acquiring a wicked set of skills and getting paid to do something that few others could do. I recalled an admonition I often heard from my good friend, General Martin Dempsey: "You don't get to be a professional just because you say you are. You actually have to understand the requirements and act the part!"

Without question, doctors are part of a noble profession. And yet many of my new healthcare colleagues appeared to describe themselves as "professional" without completely understanding the deeper requirements associated with being part of a professional body. Yes, being a member of certain professional organizations requires attendance at meetings, paying dues, and executing some administrative (or perhaps publishing) responsibilities.

But there is so much more to a profession!

I quickly saw the potential for using my lifelong interest in studying the profession of arms to help physicians make a deeper connection to their own profession of medicine. And I knew that in making that deeper connection, they'd naturally become better leaders.

The Elements of a Profession[6]

Medicine, the ministry, law, and the military have always been considered the premier historical "professions," according to social scientists. While there are certainly others (engineering, journalism, teaching, CPAs, etc.), for purpose of discussion with our doctors, I thought it best to list those four as primary, since they most precisely adhere to the agreed-upon definition of "a relatively high status occupation whose members apply abstract knowledge to solve problems in a particular field of endeavor."[7]

Over the centuries, disagreements have arisen over what constitutes a profession or which occupations should be considered professions, but much of the debate has stemmed from arguments about social status, occupational skills, and structures. If individuals believe they are part of a business, they perform and manage their organization like a business-person, with some emphasis on product or engagement but a primary focus on financial reward. If individuals truly believe they are part of a profession, however, they feel called to do something more… something special for society, especially since they have a critical skill set that obligates them in some way to the larger culture.

Because all physicians (and healthcare workers writ large) know they are special and perform a skill that no one else can perform within a community, then reinforcing their professional commitment—and the responsibilities that go along with those responsibilities—further deepen physicians' understanding of the requirements linked to leadership and leading their professional body.

A Little Background

In a treatise on the science and art of medicine, Scribonius Largus first used the word "profession" in 47 AD.[8] He noted that what made physicians unique was their commitment to compassion, benevolence, and clemency in the relief of suffering and their adherence to humanitarian values. That definition has the merit of both simplicity and directness, especially when linked with the code of Hammurabi (ca. 2000 BC), which—along with the oaths of Hippocrates and Maimonides—codified the practice of medicine as the sacred trust of all physicians.[9]

In researching what medical societies have said recently about the topic, however, I've found much more debate and discussion, and not a little confusion. While various medical societies have published documents and conducted seminars on what defines a profession, most of those have focused more on attempting to address the issues of *poor* professional behavior or "professional lapses."[10] For the PLD course, I wanted to provide a simple list that would stimulate discussion and would get participants thinking about who they were as physicians and why leadership was critical to their *professional* body of knowledge. I also wanted to compare physicians to soldiers and show why, as leaders in their field, they needed to exert some professional rigor to identify a few select elements of their profession.

I expected that by doing this, our physician leaders could use the elements they identified to create an exemplar of recommended professional behavior that could be used as part of a positive approach to leadership—different from (and more effective than) a reactive approach to disciplining unruly members of their body.

For simplicity, we showed our physicians the following five elements of a profession in hopes that it might help them better understand professional requirements and the kind of professional behavior that must flow out of them.

Five Elements of a Profession

1. Professions have a prescribed set of values and a related code of ethics.

Members of a profession live by a code of ethics. A prescribed set of both professional and personal values informs their behavior. During my initial three-week analysis of physician leadership attributes and competencies at AdventHealth, it certainly became clear that all the organization's doctors knew and practiced the Hippocratic code of ethics, commonly summarized as "Do no harm."

True professionals, however, also adhere to a prescribed set of both professional and personal values. I asked almost two dozen physicians to list their professional values; none of them could do so, although a few recalled a few values getting listed somewhere at a recent seminar or during their residency. A few, with raised eyebrows, even questioned the rationale for having and applying values in the treatment of patients or in their interactions with fellow professionals.

Like many organizations, AdventHealth does, in fact, have a prescribed list of organizational values, but not a single physician knew of their existence. In fact, none of them could name a single value on the list. When I asked several of the same physicians to name a few values that they considered personally important, "family" and "integrity" rose to the top.

Since effective leaders have to rely on values as part of a sound decision-making process, we decided to make "identifying personal and professional values" a key part of our PLD course, a subject that elicited both significant passion and terrific understanding. We'll discuss values, as part of leader attributes, in more detail later in the book.

2. Members of a profession have unmatched competence in a specified body of knowledge and skills.

3. Professions require their members to have constant and continuous formal education and training in the prescribed skills and knowledge.

These two elements are tightly linked.

Without question, the physicians working in our hospital have unique and even potent medical skills in a variety of specialty and subspecialty areas. The organization has a robust program for Continuing Medical Education (CME) related to understanding the most recent procedures, techniques, and treatment modalities. Initiatives like Physician-Nurse Rounding, Physician Shadowing, Mortality and Morbidity Reviews, and "Schwartz Center Rounding" (a program dedicated to examining the emotional reactions by healthcare teams to certain treatments and procedures) are in place and contribute to professional and personal growth in the science of healthcare.

But even the doctors themselves admitted to me a lack of education and training in the art of healthcare. They lamented that they had access to few sequential, progressive, or recurrent leadership or team-building training offerings, and little to help them understand the management of large healthcare organizations. Most of the physicians I spoke with expressed a desire to attend such professional development programs, but few of them—other than those who had decided on their own to pursue graduate education in business administration or finance—saw them as important. At the time, our organization offered little assistance to those who wanted to expand their knowledge in this part of the healthcare profession.

4. Professions have prescribed standards, and those in the profession must discipline, hold accountable, and even dismiss fellow professionals who do not adhere to the specified procedures, norms, and behaviors.

This fourth requirement of a profession often generates significant discussion among physicians. In many ways, this requirement is probably the most important element of a profession, because it has such an out-sized impact on the future of patient engagement, healthcare practice, team dynamics, and organizational behavior.

While some practices, groups, and specialties claimed they had well-understood standards for specific procedures or treatments, when pressed for documentation, or when various members of the same practice were asked the same question, it became obvious that many of the "standards" landed in the realm of personal preference. Such inconsistency can make for inefficiencies, poor coordination, and misunderstanding between physicians, practices, and most especially, patients and their families. All doctors universally know the physician training mantra of "see one, do one, teach one," but what is "seen" in the first step often skews a physician's view of profession-wide standard practices and correct procedures.

My discussions with various physicians uncovered a strong desire to generate better standards of care, whether in regard to practice, procedures, or costs. It's a hot topic. On the one hand, greater commercialization of medicine, intense competition between practices, resource constraints, and organizational dynamics all contribute to the appeal of coordinated and approved standards of practice, especially in large organizations.

On the other hand, all physicians, when discussing their profession in candid conversation, will admit to knowing one or two doctors who are allowed to "get away with" violations of medical standards. Substandard behavior by those with high volume/high cost practices, or who might garner administrative favoritism for some other reason, is sometimes excused. Doctors often dissemble when they face the requirement to discipline their own or to hold fellow physicians to professional standards. "Hey, I don't want to affect his lifestyle or his income," goes the frequent reply. But if physicians truly want to *lead* their profession—and I'm quite certain that most do—then they absolutely must make these hard calls. They have to determine which fellow professionals they need to discipline, hold accountable, and even dismiss, if necessary.

"Disciplining," of course, doesn't always mean getting someone fired or thrown out of medicine. Disciplining might also take the form of counseling, coaching, or teaching. Could a true healthcare professional address a lack of interpersonal tact in a surgery suite that went uncorrected? Could a director address the need for better "service ethos" by a physician group office manager? Might a chief medical officer tell an obese doctor who is counseling a patient on ways to prevent diabetes that there might be a reason the patient seems to pay little attention? This element of professionalism gives physicians the consent to teach, counsel, and coach others—even their peers—in regard to correct professional behavior.

5. *Members of a profession have a unique responsibility to society, based on the relatively rare and valuable skill set of those in the profession.*

Since physicians possess a unique set of essential skills that put them at the center of the healthcare profession, they have a professional responsibility to contribute beyond patient care. Physicians, in fact, must steward their profession. They must lay their hands on the rudder for change and transformation. They are in a unique position to address the various elements of the Triple Aim: increase access, reduce cost, and improve care.

A Job for Physicians Alone

No one other than physicians can do what physicians do. They have a unique skill set in healing and "fixing" people. If doctors aren't willing to contribute their professional expertise in these areas, they will essentially leave the health of their profession to those outside of the profession.

Such an idea would be abhorrent and utterly rejected in the military. It would be unthinkable. Why? Because leaders in the profession of arms know that professional responsibility and leadership *always* go hand in hand.

Both soldiers and doctors need to remember that fact. The health of the nation depends on them both holding a common commitment to safeguarding their respective, critical professions.

QUESTIONS FOR REFLECTION
AND DISCUSSION

1. Does your hospital or healthcare organization have a set of values? How are you expected to exhibit those values as part of your care for patients and in your interaction with others on the healthcare team?

2. Do you have a set of personal values? If not, why not? If so, how do you use them to make professional and personal decisions, treat patients, and live a balanced life?

3. What standards have you incorporated into your practice? Are they well known by others (physicians, clinicians, and administrators)? How do you hold others responsible for holding to those standards, and what actions are taken if you or others violate them?

4. Apply the "elements of a profession" to your practice, group, or hospital. How would you rate yourself on a 1–10 "professionalism scale" (1 = no compliance, 10 = perfect compliance)? What might you learn from others in regard to professional behavior?

WAR STORY

Private Green and Knowing Yourself

So there we were...

By February of 2008, I had been in Iraq for the first five of what would be a fifteen-month deployment. Every day brought a new adventure. The complex insurgency was in high gear, and the eleven million people who lived in northern Iraq continually demanded an improved economy and better governance.

The army uses the term "battlefield circulation" to describe a leader visiting subordinate tactical units while those units conduct combat operations. I did a lot of it, in order to gain a greater appreciation for changing conditions in the battle space.

While battlefield circulation allows a leader to look his or her leaders and soldiers in the eye, it also allows the commander to see the effectiveness of the unit, to evaluate the actions of subordinate leaders, to determine whether standards of conduct and the soldiers' morale are up to par, and to gain some firsthand snippets of intelligence regarding the enemy. All of this contributes to a better feel for current operations and how to plan future operations.

After these visits, I always returned to the headquarters with a better understanding of the enemy and with more information about the performance of our units and the quality of our soldiers. My ability to go on patrol with men thirty years my junior also helped establish trust, contributed to a positive command climate, allowed me to talk with and develop the younger leaders, and gave me insight into how we might achieve better results.

It was also fun.

My aide usually informed the unit of my arrival the night before we conducted these linkups, to learn of the kinds of missions then planned. I'd fly in a helicopter to the remote Forward Operating Base (FOB) or Combat Outpost (COP) of that unit, link up with the young officer or noncommissioned officer leading the mission, and then attempt, as best I could, to blend in with the small group of soldiers conducting the mission. Everyone knew I didn't want an entourage on these visits, so brigade and battalion commanders seldom accompanied me. It felt intimidating enough for these young soldiers to have their two-star division commander along for the ride.

On this particular day, I accompanied an infantry platoon, a group of twenty to thirty soldiers from the 101st Air Assault Division scheduled to conduct a routine patrol outside the city of Samarra. Their lieutenant, a young man of obvious tactical savvy and charismatic style, had led this small organization for quite some time. I got a positive first impression as I watched him conduct his mission briefing (communicating what would happen on the patrol) and his precombat checks (a routine where both the platoon leader and platoon sergeant check their men's equipment and preparedness for the patrol).

As he inspected his soldiers, he looked each of them in the eye, asked them some questions related to their responsibilities, and then quizzed them on how they might react to hypothetical situations. Then he asked questions about their personal life: a question or two about a wife or girlfriend, when they had last called home, whether they were getting enough sleep, etc. I could tell he had a terrific, ingrained routine. He actively engaged with those he led and did not go through the motions simply because I was watching.

I told the lieutenant I had come to observe him and his unit; I would not interfere with any of his orders during the patrol. I also told him I would provide an after-action review following the mission, as well as some information on how his unit's actions contributed to the overall situation in the north, all normal procedure in the military culture.

Taking the two-star Velcro rank off my armored vest to ensure the Iraqis we met while on patrol wouldn't see it, I then boarded the MRAP (Mine Resistant Ambush Protective vehicle). I shook hands with all the soldiers, promising not to get in their way. I also told the sergeant in charge I felt excited about seeing his men in action, because I had heard they were one of the best platoons in the brigade (something I told all the units I accompanied, to help ease their tension). Finally, I let them know I wouldn't say much during their mission but would look forward to talking with them when they were less distracted.

The next three hours found us driving to a small village, conducting a walking patrol to ensure the security of a newly refurbished Iraqi police center, talking with several citizens to assess their feelings about the changes they had seen in their village, gathering intelligence on the enemy, and having chai with a tribal sheik. Despite the uneventful patrol, it seemed clear to me this young lieutenant and his sergeant had a disciplined and well-trained team. After a quick debrief by the platoon leader, these weary infantry soldiers boarded the four MRAPs, and we began our trip back to the FOB.

I usually started talking to the soldiers on the return trip, knowing that if I formed a bond with the small team in the vehicle, I would find it much easier to talk to the entire platoon once we reached their "home" FOB. I typically threw a few questions to the soldiers in the truck—

usually six in the back, a driver, a gunner standing on a platform, and me in the front of the cab—and I prided myself on the ease with which I could get the conversation flowing.

I used my old standby to start the exchange: "So, fellas, why did you join the army?"

This question usually evoked guarded initial responses. When the men eventually did answer, most young soldiers would say things like, "Sir, I joined 'cause my dad made me" or "Sir, I joined right after 9/11" or in some cases, more swaggering replies such as, "Sir, I joined because I wanted to be a sergeant major someday!" Whatever the response, it always broke the ice.

But with this unit, my simple question triggered a wave of laughter!

"Sir," the driver finally blurted out while slapping his leg, "that's a great question. You need to ask Private Green why he joined the army."

Obviously, they had a story they wanted me to hear, and Green was the lucky trooper to tell it.

"Okay, guys," I said as I looked around the vehicle, "which one of you is Green, and why did you join the army?"

More laughter. Then a hand connected to the arm of the soldier manning the .50 caliber machine gun and standing on the platform between the driver and me came down at the side of my head. While I couldn't see his face, I could tell from the nonchalance of his wave that Green felt embarrassed to get singled out by his buddies.

"Sir, I'm up here. I'm Green." Then, after a long pause, he said with mock defiance, "And you can't make me tell you why I joined the army!"

Another burst of laughter. Obviously, this small team shared a common joke.

"Well, Green," I said with a smile, "actually, I'm your division commander, and I can make you tell me why you joined the army."

More laughter.

"Sir, here's the deal," Green said over the headset. "These guys don't want me to tell you why I joined the army; they want me to tell you what I did before I joined the army."

"Well, okay then, Green… what did you do before you joined the army?"

Another long pause. Then the answer.

"Sir, I was a male model."

The laughter now rocked the truck, so much so that the driver, a sergeant (the obvious troublemaker of the group) almost cried as he shook his head in the affirmative and gave me the thumbs-up signal. I laughed, knowing I had contributed to their bonding… but I also knew to expect a great story.

For the next several minutes, Green told me how he had worked as a male model, making a lot of money and having a lot of women chase him. In the three years since he had been "discovered" by a modeling agency at the age of nineteen, he had made well into the six figures in modeling fees. All during his story, his buddies commented on his jet-set lifestyle and reminded him that he had to introduce them to all his female model friends when the deployment ended. The conversation most certainly broke the ice. I felt like I had become one of them.

But I still hadn't seen Green's face. As we entered the FOB, the truck pulled to a stop so we could all unload and clear our weapons. I took the opportunity to issue an order: "Hey, Green, how 'bout jumping down from your position so I can see what you look like?" I said over the intercom. More laughter from the squad.

Green took off his helmet and his sunglasses, maneuvered his way from behind his machine gun, crawled down the side of the truck, and jogged up to me as I stood by the rear of the vehicle with the rest of the soldiers. Stopping and assuming the position of attention, he brought his hand up in a sharp salute. I could immediately see this young soldier certainly had the physical traits that could earn him a lot of money as a model and a lot of attention from young women. Even with a face caked with dust and streaked with sweat from our long patrol in the Iraqi heat, his wavy blond hair, chiseled chin, perfect dimples, and bright green eyes reflected a handsome specimen of manhood.

His fellow soldiers had all gathered for another round of jokes around the "clearing barrel" as we put our weapons on safe. And then I asked a question that turned them from jocular twenty-somethings into the serious professionals they had become.

"So, Green," I said, "you still haven't told me why you joined the army."

As he began his story, their demeanor changed. All of Green's soldier-buddies listened intently as he told the rest of the story. This young trooper had obviously gained the respect of his friends.

Private First Class Green had experienced the bacchanalian lifestyle of a male model for three years. He got paid what he described as an "obscene amount of money for allowing people to take pictures." He drank himself into a stupor almost every night, always surrounded by beautiful female models. It felt great early on, he said, but then he started questioning his lifestyle and his life.

"I woke up in a fancy hotel one morning after another night of binge drinking," Green said, "and I realized I had lost my soul. I looked into the bathroom mirror and I realized I didn't know who I was or what I stood for. So I decided I needed to do something more important with my life than let someone take pictures of me. Sir, it was then that I went to a recruiting station and joined the army. I haven't looked back."

I felt dumbstruck. This was the shining example of the millennial generation, a young soldier who wanted to be part of something important. Listening to his story almost brought me to tears. I knew I had to bring some humor back into the conversation or these young troopers would have to deal with a sobbing division commander.

"Okay, Green, that's a great story. But today you're running a gun truck in Northern Iraq. Are you sure you haven't looked back? How are you feeling about your decision now?"

"Hey, sir, I'm feeling pretty good about it, even on the toughest days," Green replied with a big smile. "In this organization, I know who I am.

The army taught me values... something I never had before. I'm loyal to my friends, I do my duty every day, I respect my leaders because they take care of me, and I trust my fellow soldiers because they're doing the right thing. I'm certainly making a lot less money now, so I guess I'm serving selflessly. There's honor in our cause if we do it right, my integrity is the best it's ever been, and I think my personal courage is off the chart. Especially since I'm the only one outside the armor and standing where people can shoot at me in this (censored) truck!"

Green's fellow soldiers erupted in laughter at his last remark, but they knew he had perfectly recited and given examples of all the army values found in the acronym LDRSHIP: Loyalty, Duty, Respect, Selfless Service, Honor, Integrity, and Personal Courage.

Green's story reinforced for me that values provide a base for knowing yourself, determining your actions, and leading effectively. I consider that day spent with Private First Class Green and the others in that small platoon one of the best days of my entire army career.

CHAPTER 3

Values and Great Leaders

Who comes to mind when you think of the great leaders in our nation's history? Abraham Lincoln, the selfless statesman? Harriet Tubman, a powerful voice for abolition? Dwight Eisenhower, a terrific general? Jonas Salk, a masterful researcher and virologist? Billy Graham, a powerful spiritual leader? Oprah Winfrey, an amazing entrepreneur and entertainer?

All of them, regardless of their accomplishments, have a few things in common: a strong character, an impressive presence, and a keen intellect. Leaders with these kinds of attributes have no trouble attracting loyal followers, because those followers believe the leader will consistently do the right things in the right way, regardless of the difficulty.

We need leaders with all three in contemporary healthcare.

But how do you create leaders of character, presence, and intellect? What contributes to the making of such leaders? In the profession of arms, the military uses something it calls the leadership requirements model, a paradigm based on years of research. The model centers on who the leader is and what that leader knows (attributes), and only then on what a leader does (competencies).

The army's leadership manual describes these elements in great detail. It breaks down the critical "attributes" into those three elements of character, presence, and intellect. It also shows how the application of certain characteristics of these elements brings a better understanding of how each individual can *lead* and *develop* teams to *achieve* results in the exercise of critical "competencies."[11]

My experience tells me that this model works. It is both simple and something that emerging leaders understand. Anyone who desires to be a leader in any profession can quickly understand that the elements of character, presence, and intellect contribute to developing trust with followers, and the elements of leading, developing, and achieving are required by any team to meet organizational objectives in the most effective and efficient way.

A Model for Physician Leaders

For the challenges specific to healthcare and to reflect the approach at our organization (we call it "the AdventHealth Way"), we slightly adapted the army's model to provide an excellent tool to guide our physicians on their leadership journey. We developed the following chart as a means of listing the important requirements of physician leaders. In this chapter, we'll focus on the "attributes" half of the model. As we address other aspects of leadership, we'll return to the "competencies" dimension.

The Attributes of Effective Leaders

The leader's attributes of character, presence, and intellect describe the "knowing" and "being" aspects of a leader, in contrast to the "doing" aspects connected to a leader's competencies.

The *character* of healthcare leaders is defined by what they believe

LEADER ATTRIBUTES AND COMPETENCIES

ATTRIBUTES

CHARACTER	PRESENCE	INTELLECT
⊙ Values	⊙ Bearing	⊙ Mental Agility
⊙ Empathy	⊙ Fitness	⊙ Sound Judgment
⊙ Service Ethos	⊙ Confidence in Action, Words, and Manner	⊙ Innovation
⊙ Discipline	⊙ Resilience	⊙ Interpersonal Tact
		⊙ Expertise and Practical Competence

COMPETENCIES

LEADS	DEVELOPS	ACHIEVES
⊙ Builds Trust	⊙ Creates a Positive Environment	⊙ Focused on Results
⊙ Extends Influence	⊙ Seeks Ways to Improve	
⊙ Leads by Example	⊙ Develops Others	
⊙ Communicates	⊙ Stewards of the Profession	

and the values they hold dear. Character involves how leaders view and understand others, how they apply their moral principles to decision making, and how they view their service within the profession of healthcare and the standards to which they hold themselves. Character helps leaders to determine the right thing to do, while giving them the courage and self-discipline to execute what is appropriate under all circumstances. I consider the "values" element of character so crucial that we'll spend a significant amount of this chapter focusing specifically on values, both professional and personal.

The healthcare leader's *presence* is determined by her actions, words, and the manner in which she carries herself. This presence contributes to how leaders are perceived by patients, family members, teammates, and the organization. It directly reflects their energy and, not surprisingly, their physical appearance and even their moral, intellectual, and physical fitness. The healthcare leader must exude a balance of compassion, energy, and confidence but not cockiness, even in difficult situations. A neurosurgeon wearing a Hawaiian shirt and sandals would not likely generate confidence in a patient; but if that same physician worked as a pediatric urologist, dealing exclusively with children who might think the breezy look "cool," that could be a different story (think the 1998 movie *Patch Adams*).

The healthcare leader's *intellect* is based on practiced sound judgment, informed by continuous study of interpersonal experiences and methods of innovation. While a physician's judgment is critical, equally as important might be that physician's ability to adapt or innovate, based on the situation or the environment. While patients and healthcare teammates certainly want interpersonal tact, the level of that tact might differ depending on the situation, the environment, and the trust already generated between the parties involved.

My four decades of service in the military taught me that all of these elements contribute to developing trust between the leader and those he or she leads. Trust is the coin of the realm of leadership, and when leaders understand how the application of character, presence, and intellect contribute to developing trust with their followers, they begin to understand the importance of attributes. As healthcare leaders refine and expand the elements of their character, exhibit and receive feedback on their presence, and develop the mental aspects associated with their intellect, they develop trust with those they lead—and then they can make far greater contributions to their teams and their organization.

Good leadership can and must be learned, practiced, and further developed. Growing in leadership requires self-assessment (a bit on that momentarily), definition of values, contemplating the thoughts of others on the subject of leadership, and observing other leaders as they execute their duties. It also requires continual analysis of the way proper personal interactions provide a base for leading large healthcare organizations.

How Do You Lead Yourself?

Self-reflection is a key part of the leadership journey. Anyone aspiring to be a leader will waste a lot of time if they focus on how to lead others before they have a good feel for how they lead themselves.

This declaration sometimes disappoints potential leaders, because they want to learn how to get others to follow them... quickly! Most young leaders, at least initially, have little interest in spending any time looking inward. "My followers are out there... I must go lead them!" they declare in one way or another.

But a key part of learning how to lead is learning something about the way *you* operate. Taking a good personality inventory (such as Meyers Briggs, the Core Values Index from Taylor Protocols, or as we did at AdventHealth Orlando, the AdventHealth Executive "Big Five") can reveal a great deal about who you are, how others see you (better sometimes than how you see yourself), and how you "tick." It might also provide some insight into how much energy a leader must expend in doing things he or she likes to do versus what might come as a challenge. When you combine such self-analysis with understanding the importance of character, presence, and intellect in developing a leadership style, you set yourself up for leadership success.

A Little Test

We once asked our physician leaders in the PLD class to report on the leadership attributes they observed in another healthcare professional, particularly one who serves in a leadership role. We also asked them to give examples of how the strengths or weaknesses of those attributes reinforced or detracted from the leadership competencies of the individual.

At the start of our PLD course, we asked our healthcare professionals to take a personality inventory. Some of them felt surprised by the results. (One physician reported his spouse told him she didn't understand his shock, since she had seen that side of him all their married life!) Based on what they learned from their own personality inventory, we further asked them to report on the leadership style of one individual with whom they worked and how a better understanding of their own personality mix might contribute to better teamwork and effectiveness.

We designed both tasks to challenge the physicians to build on their own qualities and attributes by observing those of others. Observing others would, in turn, allow them to better understand how leadership is involved in *every* personal interaction. Equally important, we wanted our doctors to experience, firsthand, how applying the art of leadership contributes to building effectiveness and teamwork within an organization.

Their subsequent presentations provided a foreshadowing of what we would see increasingly as the course continued over the next several months. The early formation of healthcare "teams"—doctors, clinicians, and administrators who had come together to formulate their findings and present their reports—demonstrated a previously uncharacteristic level of bonding. Barriers between physicians, nurses, and hospital executives started to break down.

We had thought it critically important to have all members of the healthcare team come together to understand how those from various "tribes" think. Most physician leadership courses do not include nurses or administrators, but by combining all three groups, we saw a collection of healthcare providers learning to trust each other while tackling tough issues together.

Prior to the class, a nurse participant who happened to be one of our more mature leaders, made an interesting sidebar comment to me. "You should have seen all the cross talk going on in preparing for this presentation," she said, smiling. "Emails and phone calls and texts! I've never seen that much exchange of communication, that much teamwork, with our doctors!"

No doubt class participants from all "tribes" felt challenged by exploring in more detail the various leadership attributes we highlighted. But also without question, our focus on "values" lit a fire for many that had not burned for a long time, if ever.

Values Determine Character

I once gave a speech to a major multinational medical supply company. The CEO and the whole C-suite would attend, as would all the managers from each nation where the company sold its product. In preparing my remarks, I asked the organizer if the company had a set of organizational values; she proudly told me the firm displayed them on its web page. I found them, to be sure, but during my presentation I also discovered that no one in the room could name a single one of them.

I wish I could say that's an anomaly. Unfortunately, I can't. I know it happens all the time, in all kinds of organizations, companies, and healthcare groups. So let's take a closer look at how organizational values and personal values assist and guide a leader.

1. Organizational Values

While it's great to have organizational values, it's even better when the individuals in that organization know them, live by them, and make decisions with those values in mind. Values lead to action, as Harry Kraemer says in his terrific book, *From Values to Action: The Four Principles of Values-Based Leadership.*

We've already seen that all professions must identify and live by a code of ethics and a prescribed set of values. For physicians to be called "professional," they must fully understand the implications of their profession's ethics and what is required in caring for others. Equally as important is to have a set of strong values to light their way. Identifying and living by a set of values goes a long way toward shaping a leader's character. In many ways, I consider values the most important of the attributes listed above. In my personal research, while I found several physicians from other medical schools and hospitals who had tackled the question of defining the right values for the profession of healthcare, I found no consensus as to what those values should be.

Why does possessing a set of values provide the required base for good leadership? Values reflect what the leader really believes and mirror what the leader sees as most important. Values guide a leader's actions during tough times, and a strong sense of personal (and perhaps organizational) values contribute to making tough decisions under difficult conditions. Frances Hesselbein of the Drucker Foundation once said, "Leadership is not a basket of tricks or skills. It is the quality and character and the value and courage of the person who is the leader." Values contribute to that quality, character, and courage.

Finally, while *possessing* a prescribed set of values is critical to the leader, *adhering* to identifiable and communicated values is also important to those being led. People want to be part of organizations led by individuals they believe in and for whom they have great respect. People tend to trust individuals who do the right things, for the right reasons. A leader's commitment to living by a set of values defines expectations and acceptable behavior for the followers. It also contributes to the trust so paramount in all leader-led relationships.

So what are values? Consider this definition:

Values are specific principles, standards, and qualities considered essential to guiding individuals and organizations. Values are instrumental in helping leaders create a common understanding of expected behavior and attaining desired standards in both simple and complex situations.

My personal values are strongly linked to the army's organizational values. Starting in basic training, every soldier learns the army's values, reinforced in every officer and NCO leadership course. Ask any person wearing the uniform about the seven army values; I guarantee you'll get a response. If you don't already know what those values are, or you don't have a soldier nearby to quiz, here's the list:

- *Loyalty* – To country, to Constitution, and to comrades, whose very lives, security, or well-being depends on my actions.

- *Duty* – To fulfill my obligation to country and organization; to ensure readiness and to continuously adhere to my oath of service.

- *Respect* – For all people, friend or foe; for established and revered codes of conduct, for those in authority, for other cultures, and for those we serve.

- *Selfless service* – Putting the welfare of the nation, the organization, and our soldiers before my own.

- *Honor* – Demonstrating an understanding of what is right and setting a positive example for others in the organization, which will contribute to the climate and morale of the force.

- *Integrity* – Doing what is right, legally and morally; being honest in word and deed, remaining committed to truths.

- *Personal courage* – To face physical or moral fear, danger, or adversity and do what is necessary; to stand firm on values, principles, and conviction.

Why did the army choose these particular values, and how are they linked to army aspirations? For one thing, they are all associated with the oath of office we took, to protect and defend the Constitution against all enemies, foreign and domestic, and to obey the orders of the president of the United States and the orders of those appointed over us. Values contribute to developing leaders of character, and honing those values contributes to the establishment of trust in life and death situations. It is also serendipitous that the letters form the acronym LDRSHIP, which every soldier can easily remember.

Each of the army values connects to organizational beliefs and desired behaviors intended to help soldiers and leaders navigate difficult terrain, surmount challenging situations, and make complex decisions. We'll discuss personal values in a moment; but do you know the values of the organization that employs you? If you work there, shouldn't your professional values nest in the principles and standards of that organization?

My own employer, AdventHealth, has developed a set of institutional values using the acronym IC-BEST (pronounced "I see best"). When I asked the members of our first PLD course to define each letter, the five administrators could do so, as could a few of the clinicians. But not one of the doctors could remember even having heard of this term. I chalked it up to a symptom of the physicians being disconnected from the rest of the healthcare team, something I had suspected many months earlier during my three-week analysis of the hospital's dynamics. In times past, a cultural separation had occurred between doctors, administrators, and clinicians.

Since I've shown you the army's core values, let me describe AdventHealth's values:

- *Integrity* – The healer's words and activities create trust, as evidenced by words that are truthful, respectful, and consistent.

- *Compassion* – The healer meets individual needs with kindness, care, and empathy.

- *Balance* – The healer displays harmony in his or her professional, personal, and community life, as well as in the mind, body, and spirit.

- *Excellence* – The healer provides care and services that are safe, reliable, and patient-centered and that drive extraordinary clinical, operational, and financial performance.

- *Stewardship* – Our hospital and our healers ensure sustainability and preeminence in patient care by responsively managing resources entrusted to us.

- *Teamwork* – We strive to create an environment that values diversity of thought and background, while encouraging individuals and patients to share their different perspectives.

One physician who saw AdventHealth's values for the first time said, "You know what I like about these values? The patient is at the center of each of them. If an executive at this hospital created this list and these definitions, then I've just changed my mind a little about who they are and what they do. Most doctors think the administration is just after the money, because that's what we see. You're opening my eyes to the fact that those who run our organization might also believe in the welfare of the patient. If shared values help us constantly remember that the patient is at the center of every equation, as leaders we ought to know what these values are all about."

Indeed. Values serve as organizational guideposts and also contribute to effective decision making.

2. Personal Values

If the difference between leadership and management depends primarily on "who you are" versus "what you do," then shouldn't each leader have a set of personal values that defines who he or she is as an individual, outside the profession or the work environment? And if that's true, then what are *your* personal values?

Whenever I pose this question to various groups, almost invariably I get silence. Nearly always, the vast majority of individuals in the room have never given much thought about their own personal values. And so I've wondered: *Is it that we don't want to share them, or is it because we haven't thought much about our personal values and haven't clearly defined what we believe in?*

Consider a few potential personal values in the chart on page 65.

Do you think that adherence to a particular value in a critical situation might change the way a leader acts in that situation? The answer is obvious, but to make the answer unforgettable, I conducted a simple exercise in one PLD class.

I asked each member of the class to choose five random values from the list. Then, after listening to a scenario, I asked them to apply their chosen values to the situation to see if the application of that value would guide their actions. All of the situations had recently occurred at AdventHealth Orlando; in addition, a medical review board had been assigned to address the inappropriate conduct associated with each case.

POTENTIAL VALUES

⊙ Service	⊙ Respect	⊙ Courage
⊙ Loyalty	⊙ Learning	⊙ Selfness
⊙ Duty	⊙ Innovation	⊙ Passion
⊙ Balance	⊙ Teamwork	⊙ Candor
⊙ Excellence	⊙ Integrity	⊙ Competency
⊙ Humor	⊙ Compassion	⊙ Curiosity
⊙ Responsiveness	⊙ Forgiveness	⊙ Greed
⊙ Caring	⊙ Kindness	⊙ Grace
⊙ Humility	⊙ Perseverance	⊙ Agility
⊙ Stewardship	⊙ Trust	⊙ Empathy
⊙ Credibility	⊙ Dignity	⊙ Accuracy

Situation #1

You are at a party and you've just met a physician from another hospital who tells you a story about treating a patient who, unbeknownst to him, was previously a patient of a physician at your hospital. This physician, who obviously does not know your longtime practice partner, begins bragging how another doctor— your partner—badly botched a surgical procedure, which he had to fix. To complicate matters, your spouse has a surgery scheduled with your partner next week. What do you do?

This scenario prompted several emotional responses. The initial responses came from those who had randomly selected "loyalty" as a value, since the scenario pointed to a conflict between loyalty to the partner and loyalty to patients. A lively discussion then ensued, centered on the issues of medical competence, adherence to professional standards, and the courage required to request an investigation into the practices of another physician. Our seminar participants reasoned that if the report about the botched surgery were true, then the operating physician (the "practice partner") had apparently not lived up to professional standards and should be confronted with his failure.

But then the discussion shifted to the talkative physician in the scenario who, by disclosing confidential information at a cocktail party, had violated hospital standards by disclosing the identity and medical condition of the patient, as well as the treatment modalities used by the other physician.

The class energetically debated the difficulties related to taking action. Would a doctor hearing another doctor talk about a surgical disaster at a party have the courage to immediately confront the first physician, labeling the casual discussion inappropriate? Could the physician discuss the issue with his practicing partner who performed the allegedly botched operation? Would the physician listening to the commentary fail to take action, but then proceed to change his spouse's scheduled operation, based on concern about his colleague's competencies?

What would your own personal values prompt *you* to do in this scenario?

Situation #2

You are in the operating room theater with a group of residents and a group of student nurses. They are scheduled to observe a well-respected and high-profit-generating physician perform a

difficult procedure. As the physician enters the suite, he asks his
team, "Would anyone mind if I told an off-color joke?"

One member of the team responds, "Doctor, we have visitors
viewing the procedure."

The surgeon replies, "Well, those who might be offended can
just close their ears." The doctor then proceeds to tell the joke,
which has overt sexual overtones.

One of the student nurses in the observation room turns to
you and says, "Is this the kind of behavior we should expect?"

One doctor who heard this story stated categorically he couldn't imagine anything like it ever happening in a reputable medical institution. Several nurses and administrators immediately replied that they had all encountered similar situations, including abusive behavior by surgeons in an operating suite.

Concern for the welfare of the patient always prevented the nurses and administrators from holding the physician to standards during the procedure (likely the right approach). But should they report the incident afterward? Our seminar participants had mixed feelings about that.

The class then engaged in a values-based discussion of whether physicians who generate high profit for the organization often get put on a longer leash, despite their less-than-respectable behavior. These comments prompted class members to return to a discussion about the elements of a profession and the application of professional standards, all driven by an adherence to values—and one of those elements requires members of the profession to discipline those who violate the group's professional standards, based on what leaders believe is best for the organization.

"Disciplining a colleague is extremely difficult," declared one physician, "but if you have a set of values to guide you and remind you what 'right' looks like, then it might be a bit easier to hold someone to a standard."

Messaging Your Values

Determining one's personal values requires much self-reflection, but it also provides a guide for balance and perspective when the time comes to weigh difficult issues. Having a firm set of values contributes to improved self-confidence and even to genuine humility in decision making.

But what if your values are personal? How will those values garner trust if those you lead don't know what values are important to you? Do you need to publicize a list, like the army and AdventHealth have done?

Take a look at the list of values again and see if you can determine what the following individuals held dear, and how those values might have affected their relationships with those they led.

Colonel Joshua Chamberlain

Chamberlain, a thirty-four-year-old former professor of rhetoric at Maine's Bowdoin University, was not the typical Union military leader in the Civil War. As the commander of the Twentieth Regiment of Infantry, Maine Volunteers, he confronted a difficult moral challenge shortly before the Battle of Gettysburg. Given the responsibility for 120 Maine volunteers who had been accused of mutiny, he was authorized to shoot them as deserters if they did not willingly join his ranks.

This solder's moral compass—the personal values guiding his actions—kept him from even considering execution. To him, human life was sacred; he was fighting for freedom and dignity, and he would never consider shooting anyone due to a difference of opinion. The 1993 movie *Gettysburg* captures a fictionalized account of Chamberlain's talk to the mutineers this way:

> I've been ordered to take you men with me. I've been told
> that if you don't come, I can shoot you. Well, you know I

won't do that. Not Maine men. I won't shoot any man who doesn't want this fight… But I will tell you this: we sure can use you. This is a different kind of army… We're here for something new. This hasn't happened much in the history of the world. We're an army going out to set other men free. This country must be free ground, all the way from here to the Pacific Ocean. A place where no man has to bow. Here we judge you by what *you* do, not by what your father was. But the idea that we all have value, you and me, we're worth something more than the dirt… I'm not asking you to come join us and fight for dirt. What we're all fighting for, in the end, is each other.

The printed word doesn't do justice to the rhetoric, and the fiction may not accurately match what he said, but Chamberlain did create a reaction. As a result of his speech, delivered under the shade of a grove of trees, 114 of the 120 mutineers changed their minds and agreed to join Chamberlain's unit. With their help, the Twentieth Maine held onto Little Round Top at Gettysburg, which many historians believe saved the day and won the battle.

What personal values do you think drove Chamberlain?

Gordon Gekko

Now think of a different character, featured in the 1987 movie *Wall Street*. Michael Douglas, who won an Academy Award for his portrayal of Gordon Gekko, delivers his famous "greed is good" monologue to a roomful of stockholders and executive officers, influencing the likes of his protégé, Charlie Sheen, and others. He says:

Teldar Paper has thirty-three different vice presidents, each earning over two hundred thousand dollars a year. Now, I have spent the last two months analyzing what all these guys do, and I still can't figure it out. One thing I do know is that our paper company lost 110 million dollars last year, and I'll bet that half of that was spent in all the paperwork going back and forth between all these vice presidents. The new law of evolution in corporate America seems to be survival of the unfittest. Well, in my book you either do it right or you get eliminated.

In the last seven deals that I've been involved with, there were 2.5 million stockholders who have made a pretax profit of twelve billion dollars. Thank you.

I am not a destroyer of companies. I am a liberator of them!

The point is, ladies and gentlemen, that greed—for lack of a better word—is good. Greed is right. Greed works. Greed clarifies, cuts through, and captures the essence of the evolutionary spirit. Greed, in all of its forms—greed for life, for money, for love, knowledge—has marked the upward surge of mankind. And greed—you mark my words—will not only save Teldar Paper, but that other malfunctioning corporation called the USA.

In contrast to Chamberlain, Gekko is a self-interested mercenary, using others for his purpose of generating more deals and more wealth. He is certainly an "influential" leader, but a consummately toxic one (see page 95). He comes to an unhappy end in the movie, facing criminal charges and jail time, but his downfall occurs only after he has destroyed countless lives and companies with his particular set of values.

What personal values do you think drove Gekko?

Chamberlain was able to influence others as a result of his ability to articulate his beliefs: honesty, integrity, respect, loyalty, and trust. Gekko's values were well-represented by his mantra "greed is good," setting the conditions for his eventual self-destruction.

How you live, the words you speak, and the way you act as a leader reveal your true beliefs. And your real beliefs will lead you down a particular path, whether for good or for ill.

A Progress Report

After our classroom discussion of values, we gave our PLD healthcare leaders a simple assignment:

1. Develop and define five personal values and come prepared at the next class to discuss how you personify each one in your personal life.

2. Observe some aspect of the identified "AdventHealth Values" (Integrity, Compassion, Balance, Excellence, Stewardship, and Trust) and report on ways they contribute to decision making within the organization.

3. Observe and prepare to discuss any values-based dilemmas that you may face during the month.

One accomplished surgeon chosen to present his team's report—a doctor who got three totally different responses when he asked the three people closest to him to identify his values—asked permission to give an individual report. He spoke to the group from the heart; the exercise clearly had a profound effect on him.

"At first, I laughed about it," he said, referring to the three radically different responses he'd received. But the laughter didn't last long:

> Then I realized that all of them were seeing a different side of who I am, which probably meant I wasn't being true to myself. I thought about that for several days; it really bugged me. It concerned me to know that if I'm asked to make decisions regarding a difficult situation in either my professional or personal life, based on my values and what I truly believe in, I'll likely just blow in the wind. I won't rely on my beliefs as to what is right or wrong.
>
> This last week, I took some time every night to think and pray about this, and I've come up with five values that really mean a lot to me and that I'm comfortable with. I showed my wife these values and shared with her my thoughts. We got into a much deeper conversation than I had expected. She told me she thinks that because of this little drill, I'll likely be a much better person. During that exchange, she actually told me that in the last few years, she thought I was losing my way; I had gotten so busy and had stopped thinking about the reasons I once had for wanting to be a doctor. Since that conversation, I've really come to peace with all this.
>
> What's really interesting is that I've shared these five values with the members of my practice. We had a great conversation about them, and over the last two weeks, I've really focused on making decisions based on those values. It's amazing how much more confident I am in my actions and how the members of my team seem to know which way I'll go on an issue, even before I tell them what to do. In the short period of time since I made a decision based on this new set of defined values, I've detected better

communication with patients and their families and a reduction in the amount of "drama" going on within the practice.

While I'm not going to share my personal values with you today, I do want you to know that I have them firmly planted in my heart. Funny thing is, some of the other physicians in my practice are using the same sheet of "value words" to think about their personal values, too. We're even considering complementing the AdventHealth values with our own "group" values.

Before this doctor gave his personal report to the whole class, he had approached me privately to say, with deep concern in his voice, "Mark, three people who know me well are seeing three different people in me. I'm not sure I'm being true to myself. I think I have a lot of work to do in building a values base for good leadership."

I replied that if his discovery troubled him, he was on his way and that he would be just fine.

What about you?

A strong set of values, coupled with confidence in action and greater interpersonal tact, will certainly build trust and help to create a more positive organizational environment. Self-discipline, linked to innovative thinking, will also contribute to better results in any organization. In fact, a combination of *any* of the attributes listed earlier will always contribute to leadership success.

But whatever you do, *don't forget your values.* Let them do the work that they're marvelously equipped to do.

QUESTIONS FOR REFLECTION
AND DISCUSSION

1. How would you describe your personal leadership strengths and weaknesses?

2. Are you an introvert who doesn't like to engage with large groups? Or an extrovert who enjoys being in large groups? How do you apply your personality when dealing with others as you lead?

3. Does your organization have a set of institutional values? If so, what are they, and how are they applied in decision making?

4. Do you have a set of personal values that reflect your experiences, your background, and what you hold dear? If not, pick five from the chart in this chapter that resonate with you, and attempt to apply them to situations in your life to determine how your decisions are affected. If so, how do they affect your leadership and your decision making?

5. In reviewing "attributes," which of the character, presence, and intellect elements do you see as your strengths? Which ones do you think you need to further develop?

WAR STORY

Lessons for a Young Lieutenant

So there we were…

In late fall of 1975, I was a brand new second lieutenant, reporting to my first army unit. Wearing my sharp dress green uniform, with one ribbon above my left breast pocket, I waited in the outer office to see the lieutenant colonel who commanded this armor battalion in Schweinfurt, Germany. The first lieutenant adjutant guarding the perimeter seemed so worldly. *He must be in his mid-twenties!* I thought.

"Well, Lieutenant Hertling," the adjutant asked, looking up from his papers, "are you ready to be a tank platoon leader?"

"Yes, sir," I replied, not knowing what demands would present themselves in my first job. I had just arrived in Germany that morning, at the height of the Cold War. After six months of training with tanks at Fort Knox following my graduation from the military academy, I felt excited about the challenges I would face… but also nervous.

"Well," the more experienced lieutenant said, "I'm sure the boss might throw some things your way."

75

As he spoke, the battalion commander—a man responsible for more than eight hundred soldiers and fifty-four tanks but who looked younger than his thirty-five years—appeared in his office doorway. "So, you're Lieutenant Hertling," he said with a big smile. "Come on in, and let's talk." *This couldn't possibly be the man who had so much responsibility*, I thought. He seemed too energetic, too friendly.

Standing at attention in front of the battalion commander's desk, I fielded all sorts of questions about my training at the Armor Officer Basic Course, my degree from West Point (he'd also graduated from West Point), my family, why I chose Germany as my first assignment, why I chose armor as my branch, and many other topics I no longer recall. He made an instant positive impression.

Then, his tone changed and he became serious. "Lieutenant Hertling," he said, "you've been assigned to a front line unit. The Soviets could come across the border at any time, and we have to be ready if they do. Every day. Here's your mission for today: I want you to meet the soldiers in your tank platoon, and then I want you to coordinate your platoon's movement out to the place where you will fight. We call it the General Defensive Position, or GDP. I'll meet you there tomorrow morning at 0600 hours. You'll brief me on your maintenance and personnel status and how you will fight the Soviets, should they attack your position. Any questions?"

"Ummm… no, sir," I replied. "You'll be out there at six *tomorrow* morning?"

He subdued a smile and answered, "That's right… first thing tomorrow. I know you'll be ready. You'd better get moving, lieutenant." I saluted, did a sharp about-face, and walked quickly past the smirking adjutant.

I headed to Alpha Company.

The company commander, an older Vietnam veteran, greeted me as I arrived. He pulled me into his office and asked if I had received a mission from the battalion commander. He then explained this was the colonel's "rite of passage for all newbies." It was also my chance to make a great first impression. He then told me I would be leading First Platoon and that my platoon sergeant would help me accomplish the mission.

Minutes later, the platoon sergeant arrived at the orderly room and bellowed, "I hear there's a new lieutenant who's going to lead First Platoon." I introduced myself, we shook hands, and he told me to follow him to the motor pool. As we walked, we discussed the mission.

"Here's what we need to do, lieutenant," he said. "In a few minutes, I'm going to introduce you to the men. You'll want to issue them a warning order, telling them what we'll be doing for the next few days, to get them moving. Then you and I will conduct a little recon (reconnaissance) to our GDP. It's about forty miles from here, so we'll have time to talk on the way."

The platoon sergeant, a grizzled old noncommissioned officer, seemed about twenty years my senior. He wore the patch of a combat veteran; I later found out he had served two tours as a tanker in Vietnam. He had been wounded in action and had performed various acts of heroism. Now he'd been saddled with training a new lieutenant, a "newbie."

He asked if I wanted a cup of coffee and if I took it with cream and sugar. "That would be great, sergeant. Thanks," I said.

"Okay, this is your first lesson," he responded, with mock patience. "We drink our coffee black in First Platoon. Putting cream and sugar in it means you're taking a break, and we don't have time for any breaks... we have a lot of work to do. Plus, when we're in the field, we don't have time to carry a lot of cream and sugar in our tanks. So you might as well get used to it. Our soldiers don't want to see their lieutenant being a wimp and drinking his coffee with cream and sugar!"

I didn't know if he was kidding, so I quickly said, "Black will be fine."

After coffee, we went to meet the platoon. The platoon sergeant formed the men, told them who I was, and watched as I gave my first remarks to this group of nineteen young soldiers. I told them of our mission and that we'd be in the field for a few days. The platoon sergeant then directed me to the motor pool, to our five parked tanks. The men, while friendly enough, seemed unimpressed with their new leader. But the tanks still looked intimidating.

Within an hour, we headed off in the platoon sergeant's car, a "hooptie," as the soldiers all called the beat-up, run-down vehicle he had purchased in Germany. We sped along toward our GDP, along the West German–Czechoslovakian border. During the hour-long trip, I received more leadership advice than I had received in all four years at West Point.

"Okay, Lieutenant Hertling," the platoon sergeant started, "you're now *my* platoon leader. I take a great deal of pride in how *our* platoon, and how *my* lieutenant, perform. You did pretty good when you first addressed the men, but I'm going to give you a few tips on how you may want to handle this mission."

With that, the monologue began. When I addressed the men, he noticed I talked to them as a group. "Great leaders focus on the individuals, not on the size of the platoon," he said. "Leadership is one person at a time. You may see a platoon of nineteen soldiers standing in front of you, but you'll do much better if you see each individual soldier, and you know his strengths, weaknesses, and what motivates each one."

He then told me details about each soldier: his personality, his wife or girlfriend, what motivated him, the things he might do to get in trouble, his background, the man's potential for advancement or his likelihood of winding up in jail. He advised me to take time over the next twenty-four hours to get to know each soldier and to take his thoughts into consideration.

"And by the way," he said, "don't mention that you just graduated from West Point. They all know you went there and that could be a good or a bad thing. How they will look at that will depend on how you perform as their leader. Most of these guys haven't finished high school, but they all know their job and they want to tell you about it. Be humble, listen to them, learn what they do, let them know what your standards are and what we have to accomplish as a team, and then hold them responsible for

their end of the deal. If you do that, you'll be more than you appear to be...
and that's a whole lot better than showing them your West Point ring."

We arrived at the GDP and walked the ground for several hours while
talking more about leadership. This platoon sergeant took responsibility
for growing me as a leader in his organization, because that's what great
leaders do.

As we drove back to Schweinfurt, he mentioned he thought we
should "roll the platoon" out the gate that night to come to this location.
The traffic would lessen after dark, he explained, I could take the time
to get to know "my" soldiers as we bivouacked, and we'd be positioned
for the colonel when he arrived at six a.m.

"Leaders are never late," he declared. "That shows a lack of respect
for other people."

I won't go into the details of what happened over the next few days.
Suffice it to say, I got off on the right foot in my army career because of
my first platoon sergeant. He taught me that leaders know who they are,
present themselves well, and interact with one person at a time. And he
taught me, by word and example, that good leaders do all these things
to grow others in the organization.

CHAPTER 4

Dyadic Leadership:
Leading One before Many

During four decades of commanding and leading organizations ranging in size from a nineteen-soldier tank platoon to a 100,000+ soldier multinational task force in Northern Iraq, I always faced challenges. At each level of leadership, from lieutenant to three-star general, I faced difficult tasks, complex situations, challenging personalities, and diverse approaches to getting the job done.

But throughout those years, one guiding principle never changed. To lead, you first need to get buy-in, one follower at a time: up (superiors), down (subordinates), and sideways (peers).

So it's time to turn up the rheostat. The time has come to introduce the variable that makes leading so hard. How does a leader engage and influence *only one other individual*? That's dyadic leadership, and it's as difficult as it is crucial.

One Before Many

Sometimes "followers" come as individuals, or more commonly in groups, teams, or large organizations. The number of those followers and their location in the organization will vary. But before I could lead a tank platoon on a mission, I first had to influence the platoon sergeant (he would certainly influence me), and then I had to start influencing each individual soldier on the team. As commander of US Army, Europe, I had to influence colleagues, international partners, and subordinates, all while being influenced by them, to accomplish a variety of complex tasks.

Leading and accomplishing goals and organizational objectives always start by understanding just one other person's point of view. Once the leader gains that understanding, he or she can determine which influence technique to use. And after the leader understands that one individual, and then all the others, and recognizes what it will take to lead them, the leader then must perform several other related tasks. He or she must communicate the vision, publicize the standards, hold followers accountable, and push toward and accomplish the objective. If a leader can first master the techniques and understand the intricacies associated with influencing others in a one-on-one relationship, then that same leader, with more time, experience, increased responsibility, and luck, can learn to effectively lead and influence an organization of any size to reach a variety of objectives.

That's what we need physicians to do in healthcare.

In the healthcare environment, every physician interacts one-on-one with a variety of patients, patient family members, other health-care professionals and colleagues, and administrators. Each encounter requires a unique approach, and in each one the physician leader must understand what motivates the other and decide on a blend of influence techniques. Many aspiring leaders, however, think and talk only about what *they* believe is important, without considering the other's motivation or point of view. That's not good leadership, and it doesn't contribute to a high-performing organization.

Leadership requires competency and confidence (two of the attributes discussed earlier), which all physicians have in spades. But leadership also requires humility, interpersonal tact, empathy, and great communication skills. We don't always find these attributes in individuals who are highly degreed, well trained, accomplished, and busy... like a general or a doctor![12]

While most generals receive training specifically designed to put their egos in check (and some don't do so well in that training), few physicians get such training. We school them to believe they have the right answer, the right diagnosis, the right approach, and the right prescription for every medical situation. In most cases, they really do have those correct answers; doctors are, after all, experts in the human body and in medicine.

When they communicate their medical expertise to a patient, however, physicians sometimes unfortunately fail to consider what motivates the person who has to act on the information. If the doctor doesn't lead—which requires empathy and the exercise of some form of influence to encourage the patient to follow through on the prescribed plan of action—a patient might not completely understand the requirements for healing and recovery, or he or she might not see the need for following the doctor's advice. While poor outcomes often get chalked up to bad communication or "poor bedside manner," they might also be termed poor leadership. The inability of a physician to "lead," as defined by understanding another's motivations and then using the correct influence techniques to accomplish some stated objective, might contribute to a patient's extended hospital stays, improper care, incorrect use of prescribed medication, and excessive repeat visits to an emergency department. Certainly, poor physician leadership reflects badly on the hospital or clinic where the physician practices.

The Inspector General

In the army, an inspector general (IG) ensures that organizations operate in compliance with established policies and encourages them to strive to improve their effectiveness. This model goes back to the Revolutionary War, when George Washington picked the first inspector general (Prussian immigrant Baron Wilhelm von Steuben) to help determine the standards of training of American troops at Valley Forge. While most citizens today see inspectors general investigating the wrongdoings of government officials, IGs also provide many other services. IGs routinely conduct Command Climate Surveys to determine the effectiveness of organizations and the quality of leaders within those organizations.

Healthcare is increasingly looking to find what defines good hospital performance and what defines quality in healthcare leaders. Since 2005, the federal government has used a survey to evaluate hospital performance and care, called HCAHPS (Hospital Consumer Assessment of Healthcare Providers and System). HCAHPS evaluates patient perspectives on nine key topics: communication with doctors; communication with nurses; responsiveness of hospital staff; pain management; communication about medicines; discharge information; cleanliness of the hospital environment; quietness of the hospital environment; and transition of care. Prior to HCAHPS, no national standard existed for collecting or publicly reporting patients' perspectives of care. The system now provides helpful data that enables valid comparisons to be made across all hospitals in the country.

This survey instrument has created incentives for hospitals to improve their quality of healthcare while enhancing public accountability. In effect, HCAHPS measures the individual performance of physicians, but it also measures indicators of how a healthcare organization addresses key areas related to the Triple Aim of increased access, reduced costs, and improved care. Can you guess the area that has the lowest rated scores of all the areas measured by HCAHPS in most hospitals across the country? The current lowest scores typically come in the "physician communication" area.

I see the HCAHPS as a "healthcare IG" inspection. I also know that many people dispute the findings of an IG investigation when those results indicate the existence of problems. It is human nature to defend your own space and your own organization, especially when someone tells you things you don't want to hear. In discussing the "physician communication" HCAHPS scores, many doctors quickly point out why these scores do not accurately reflect the real situation and why second- and third-order reasons can explain ratings that fall consistently below the rest of the nine evaluated areas. While physicians can present interesting arguments, however, those opinions usually are irrelevant. Often, doctors may not be "seeing themselves," as the Chinese military philosopher Sun Tzu said. And so instead of finding ways to address and fix the problem, some physicians instead make excuses.

When physicians grow as leaders, they grow both personally and professionally. Effective physician leaders almost inevitably help their hospitals improve in the "physician communication" survey results, which contributes to greater public accountability, improved hospital ratings, and better payment for physicians. And when physicians learn how to more effectively lead, they also learn skills that will help them to become agents of change in the wider world of healthcare.

It's important for physicians to develop and use ever-improving skills with individual patients, patient family members, and other members of the healthcare team in order to address individual medical issues. But it's also vital that they practice and hone these skills for the time when they assume positions of increasing responsibility as leaders in healthcare teams and organizations. Most physicians want a seat at the table to influence healthcare's future. An admirable desire! Some physicians, however, wrongly believe their medical expertise alone qualifies them to sit at that table. To gain and keep a seat at the table, physician leaders must understand that they need empathy, the ability to use various influence techniques, and the skill to employ good communication skills that can equip them to interact effectively with both patients and those who are deciding healthcare's future.

Physicians who desire to be great healthcare leaders need to learn and constantly improve their dyadic leadership skills for the time they acquire a seat at the executive table of healthcare. Learning and practicing great bedside manners lead to better table manners when physician leaders assume higher positions of organizational leadership.

To improve communication—to affect the Triple Aim—healthcare leaders must understand other's motivations and then use some appropriate form of influence in every interaction. Improved communication, understanding the other person, getting a read for the circumstances, and using appropriate methods of influence can all contribute to getting things done.

The Role of Influence

"I'm really interested in what we're going to learn about dyadic leadership," one doctor said to me before a class on the topic, "because in a hospital environment, I'm not sure we can apply most of the things you're going to teach us."

"What makes you think that?" I asked.

"Well, you have a military background and you're a general," he said. "You're used to ordering people around and making things happen. While I'd like to learn how to do that effectively, I don't think the hierarchical approach will work in healthcare."

"Yes," I replied, laughing. "We'll discuss compliance or directive leadership, which is what you're talking about, because it's on one end of a wide influence spectrum. And yes, in the military, we sometimes have to give orders that require immediate and unquestioned obedience. But we use that style only about 2 percent of the time! And it's reserved exclusively for situations where a specific reaction must occur, without question or debate. Sort of like when a surgeon demands 'scalpel!' in the operating room, and you expect to immediately receive that instrument in your open hand."

To lead well, a leader must be able to exert effective influence over others, which requires knowing what kinds of influence techniques work best with specific people in particular situations. The choice of influence technique always depends on several factors: the situation, what motivates the other person, the level of trust the leader has established, and the communication methods the leader feels most comfortable using.

Influence requires caring about what others think, having compassion for their motivations, and then including them in decision making. It's about getting buy-in, regardless of whether the leader has a powerful personality. It's more about showing that the leader cares and wants to ensure that the best idea wins, for the good of the organization.

The Influence Spectrum

Influence has a lot to do with a focus on developing one's character, one's presence, and one's intellect as a means of becoming a better leader (chart on page 54). These attributes define who the leader *is*. Each individual may be strong or weak in one or another of these elements, but each requires attention. That's what it takes for a leader to develop his or her personal leadership toolbox.

All of these attributes contribute to what the leader will be asked to *do*: lead, develop, and achieve. I've listed these elements on the chart under the category of competencies.

If a leader were asked to take over a dysfunctional organization that desperately needed to "build trust," that leader likely would need a strong set of values, sound judgment in developing processes, and great expertise in personal psychology. If the physician leader were asked to "develop others" in the organization, the requirements likely would change—perhaps to a need for unique intellectual bearing, an empathy for each person's growth, or an innovative way of coaching and mentoring.

Leading, developing, and achieving are all action verbs. They require some form of interaction with another individual (or group of individuals). Each of these leader competencies requires some type or blend of influence techniques; the leader must determine which one(s) might provide the best outcome. Remember, leadership is an art, not an exact science. Determining the right influence or the right blend of influence methods requires deep analysis of several variables: the strengths and weaknesses of the leader's attributes, the motivations of the follower, the specific situation, the time requirements associated with getting the job done, and the goals of the leader. What the leader wants to *do* depends on his or her style, the audience, and the objective. A leader might apply several methods of influence:[13]

Pressure or directive method

Leaders use this method to express a specific demand, with either an implied or explicit suspense. For a trained soldier, hearing the words "hit the dirt, incoming!" from a person in authority or someone familiar with the sound of incoming artillery usually generates an immediate response. No one needs to discuss a suspense date or how fast the person should fall to the ground. For a trained healthcare professional, the announcement of a code over a loudspeaker generates a similar response.

Authoritative request

With this influence technique, someone in a position of authority uses that authority as a basis for a request. It usually involves specific requirements and completion deadlines, with negative repercussions for unmet achievement. "If your son cuts his cast off one more time before the end of this month, his arm will not heal and he'll never throw a baseball again," the orthopedic surgeon might say. In the army, anything a drill sergeant says to a new trainee is an example of an authoritative request.

Exchange

In this technique, the leader provides some desired action or item in trade for compliance with the request. A cardiovascular surgeon might offer a series of lectures on heart disease in exchange for the donation of money for a new CV clinic. A commander might promise a four-day pass for all those who contribute to passing a maintenance inspection.

A personal appeal

This method might be used when a leader asks a follower to comply with a request based on loyalty or friendship, while at the same time knowing it is the right thing to do. A family practice physician who knows a patient is not taking prescribed medication might tell the individual he feels concerned that his failure to comply could result in added complications, and that the patient will need to find another doctor if he continues to ignore the prescription. A colonel might remind his troops that he is asking them to accomplish a tough mission because of their oath of allegiance to defend the country.

Rational persuasion

This technique requires the leader to provide data or logical arguments as to how the request relates to the objective. In this method, the leader must provide evidence in the form of research findings, strong anecdotes, or illustrations of what has worked in the past. All armor officers know the maxim, "Don't use tanks in urban environments without the support of infantry," because the directive has behind it a host of data, historical anecdotes, and negative illustrations that describe what happens when someone violates this rule. "Don't smoke, as doing so has a high correlation to lung cancer," is a similar tenet, also with death cited as a frequent result of ignoring the guideline.

Collaboration

This method involves the leader cooperating in the accomplishment of the goals, telling those led that the leader is prepared to step in at any time to help accomplish the objectives or resolve any problem that arises. In this method, the leader must be careful to not get overly involved, as that would negatively influence the relationship and the accomplishment of the task.

Inspirational appeal

This method has the leader creating excitement, gaining enthusiasm for the request by arousing emotion and building conviction. A healthcare leader might generate excitement in a team tackling a difficult medical problem by suggesting that finding the right solution could change the course of global treatment. A sergeant might suggest to his squad how accomplishing a specific part of the mission might contribute to the entire army winning the war.

Participation or consensus building

Here, the leader asks the follower to take part in the planning as well as the problem solving process. The act of determining the right solutions and reaching a specific goal leads to an increased sense of ownership of the action, from beginning to end. This influence method allows all members of the team to believe they have contributed to the successful accomplishment of the objectives. A physician allowing a patient, the patient's family, and the other members of the healthcare team to contribute ideas to the best treatment scenario is an example. Even if the doctor already knows the best method and can prescribe the approach without any additional input, participation becomes a powerful tool in getting the patient to adhere to the recommended medical treatment.

While most physicians likely have used one or more of these methods (or have been "victims" of others using them), many have not considered them as tools of leadership. One key aspect of exerting influence involves determining the right influence method(s) to use with the right person at the right time. This requires understanding the motivations of the follower, analyzing the situation, and doing whatever seems required to get the job done. This kind of leadership is truly an art.

We have an expression in the military whenever we're developing plans: "The enemy gets a vote!" Any specific technique or any blend of techniques might work in any given situation, but in order to feel more assured of success in using these techniques, the leader has to understand the motivations of those being led (especially if they're acting like an enemy).

Understanding Motivation

Leadership is who you are and how you engage with other individuals to accomplish a task. In any human interaction, a good leader has to understand that the other person should always get a vote on how to achieve some goal or reach some objective.

I have seen phenomenal leaders placed in situations where they did not consider the motivation of their followers; they failed miserably. At other times, I've watched good leaders, who took extra time to understand the members of their team, achieve unparalleled success. Individuals might possess all the attributes of character, presence, and intellect described in our chart, but if they do not know how to build trust, extend influence, lead by example, and communicate goals, they won't be able to effectively lead. In each of these competencies, the view of the other person, the one being led, must be considered.

There is no such thing as external motivation. Whenever I hear someone say, "I'll motivate this group to accomplish the mission," I think, *Good luck with that*. In fact, all motivation is intrinsic. Great leaders realize that they can attempt to understand the motivation of another, and then attempt to influence the person by engaging that motivation, only if they take the time to know that individual and discover what lights his or her fire.

So what motivates healthcare professionals? I've informally investigated the question and have to admit I've received a few surprises. Consider the most common responses I've heard:

- *A desire to help others*
- *A pleasant work environment*
- *A sense of accomplishment*
- *Scientific discovery and progress*
- *Money*
- *The opportunity to do work that results in favorable outcomes*
- *A desire to be part of a healing team*

All of the healthcare professionals I've spoken to about this agreed they had internalized one or more of the motivations listed. All of them said they take pride in being part of the healthcare profession. While a few of them mentioned "making a lot of money" as a motivator, that wasn't close to being the top motivator.

But then I posed another question: "What motivates your patients?"

"Getting well," they all replied. And that was it. I waited for more responses, to no avail. I got nothing more.

Do we really think that *every* patient who comes into *every* hospital or who comes into *every* appointment has only one motivation for coming, and that's "to get well"? *Really?*

If physician leaders don't know what motivates their patients, how can they lead them to better health? Without better understanding their individual fears and what is happening uniquely to them, how can they motivate them to get well or stay on their medication?

Will the effort to better understand a patient's motivation take a lot of time? Maybe. But we have a saying in the army: "There's never enough time to do it right, but there's always enough time to do it over."

Picturing Motivation

The terrific movie *The Blind Side*, starring Sandra Bullock and Quinton Aaron, portrayed the life of Michael Oher, an African-American youth born to a drug addict mother and a father in and out of prison. Bullock plays Leigh Anne Tuohy, the woman who became his adoptive mother during his high school years.

Michael received little attention during his childhood and attended eleven different schools during his first nine years as a student. Late in high school, the Tuohy family adopted him after becoming familiar with his difficult childhood. Oher began playing high school football and went on to grab All-American honors at the University of Mississippi. He eventually played for the Baltimore Ravens in the NFL, making it to the Super Bowl.

One scene depicts Michael at one of his first high school football practices. While he has impressive size, he lacks the skills or the instincts to bring his bulk to bear and to contribute to the team's performance. His coach repeatedly gives direction in football-ese, but the coach can't seem to influence Oher's action. At that point, Bullock walks out onto the field to speak directly to her son. She compares blocking and protecting the quarterback to Oher's motivation to protect his newly adopted family.

Unlike the coach, she doesn't yell or embarrass him. Oher immediately understands the connection between what the team has asked him to do and his desire to protect his two new siblings. At that moment, he begins to execute and plays flawlessly.

Bullock walks off the field, casually addressing the coach with the line, "You should get to know your players, Bert."

Or consider another clip from the movie *Jerry Maguire*. In the famous "show me the money" scene, Cuba Gooding Jr. implores his agent, played by Tom Cruise, to get the best contract possible from the Arizona Cardinals. Gooding explains that his wife likes him, his children like him, and his family is important to him… but Cruise will win him over as a client only when he shows Gooding the money. Money wasn't the real motivator, however; the real motivator was a desire to feel respected for his talents, his dedication, and his loyalty to the team.

One player felt motivated by a desire to protect his new family. Another player used the term "show me the money" to voice his inner desire for respect.

You really do need to get to know your players!

A Few Interaction Tips

To effectively lead, physician leaders must employ empathy to get a feel for what's on a patient's mind, even though it may have nothing to do with the injury or malady. They must do this with humility, along with displaying competence and confidence, because even though they might already know the best treatment to prescribe, they need to give the patient an opportunity to feed them additional information. Only after doing all these things should the physician leader give the patient medical advice or a prescription.

While that's all true, never forget that the devil is in the details! Consider a few more tools that good leaders keep in their toolbox.

In all communication, good leaders remember the ratio of ears to mouth. Since they have two ears and only one mouth, they need to listen twice as much as they speak. And because listening is an active skill, leaders also must use their other senses to supplement their listening skills. They must use their eyes to see if the follower—the patient, or anyone else they are leading—truly comprehends what they say. As they communicate, it's important to remain upbeat and passionate, making every effort to overcome the follower's anxiety or fear. Leaders *can't* be passive; they *must* actively use the tools in their leadership toolbox to exert their influence to arrive at a good outcome for everyone.

Leaders generate trust through their character and their presence—and remember, trust is the key contributor to leadership. Then, leaders extend their influence through understanding the situation and the individual they want to lead, which requires the application of their intellect and awareness. Until a leader has all that working together, no one can effectively lead, develop, or achieve the best results.

Toxic Leaders

A caveat attaches to applying influence methods. For these techniques to work for the good of the organization, the leader must be authentic *and* the leader must always have the follower's best interests at stake. A selfish agenda or a leader using these techniques in either a real or a perceived self-serving manner will yield, at best, compliance. And that will not contribute to building a strong team that can tackle any challenge and meet any organizational objective.

If a leader attempts to *manipulate* versus *understand* the follower's motivation, it will usually result in negative outcomes for the entire organization. A leader who does this might even be described as "toxic."

The military has wrestled with the term "toxic leadership" over the past few years, but those who possess the characteristics linked to this style are present in any professional organization. Toxic leadership is a combination of self-centered attitudes and behaviors that do not take into account the motivation of others. The application of this leadership style will always have adverse effects on subordinates, the organization, and the targeted goals. For that reason, it is important to describe a toxic leader so organizations can be on the lookout for those exhibiting toxic traits.

Toxic leaders lack concern for others or for the organization's culture. They have an inflated sense of self-worth and believe their way to approach a task is always better than any other approach. Toxic leaders place their own interests—usually associated with the desire for more power, better title, or rapid career advancement—above the goals of the organization. They are masters in using the various influence techniques to their advantage, but usually they are quite manipulative, coercive, deceptive, and intimidating when employing them. They rarely consider what motivates others.

Toxic leaders are at their most disruptive when they use their positional power to influence. Their actions are sure to undermine the will, the initiative, and the potential of their followers to contribute to organizational goals.

While you can't fix all toxic leaders, you can always uphold the standards of the healthcare profession. Growing into the increased responsibilities that come with being a true leader in the profession means physician leaders need to contribute to the climate of the organization. That means understanding the motivations of toxic leaders, along with a responsibility to attempt to influence them to adhere to designated professional standards. If a toxic leader refuses to be influenced—if he or she refuses to get "fixed"—then more disciplinary action may be required.

Leadership is more than understanding those who are pure in spirit and thought. It requires more than simply communicating organizational goals to help a team reach a stated objective. Leadership is also recognizing that, sometimes, individuals have motivations that run counter to the organization's objectives. Leaders have a key role to play in helping to adjust those motivations, or helping rid the organization of the individuals who hinder it from accomplishing its mission.

Showing someone the door is often one of the hardest things leaders are asked to do. But it may be one of the most critical needs an organization has to stay on track and be true to its mission. It's one of those nuances not included in the leadership definition featured on the chart.

QUESTIONS FOR REFLECTION
AND DISCUSSION

1. Think through five leadership interactions you've had this week. What influence techniques did you apply? Were they the right ones for the situation, or could you have done things differently?

2. Of the five interactions you used for question 1, what do you think motivated the other individual? Were you aware of these motivations before you attempted to exert influence? Did your use of a particular influence technique take that into consideration?

3. What ways do you build trust with others (patients, staff, coworkers)?

4. Are there toxic leaders in your organization? If so, how do you influence them so that they might better contribute to the organization's goals?

WAR STORY

Leaders Don't Have the Right
to Have a Bad Day

So there we were...

As a major (two-star) general in 2007–2008, I commanded the First Armored Division and Multinational Division-North in Iraq. Our force consisted of thirty thousand American soldiers and five divisions of Iraqi Security Forces. Our job centered on security for the sprawling area north of Baghdad, which encompassed five of the nine largest cities in Iraq, including the city of Mosul. Our combined U.S.-Iraqi forces made tremendous progress during the famous "surge," which quelled for a time the insurgency that threatened to overwhelm a fledgling Iraqi government.

Our units had focused on several objectives, one of them to help the Iraqis improve their capabilities in provincial government. To this end, we needed to help Iraqi businesses open and broaden their economic initiatives. We also wanted to grow and support the fledgling Iraqi army and police as they addressed internal and external security requirements in their cities and on their borders with Turkey, Syria, and Iran. And in addition to all of these tasks, we also continued to plan and conduct combat operations.

As a leader, I knew I had to build trust and confidence with our Iraqi governmental, business, and security force partners. This role required "leading up," or attempting to positively persuade and influence those over whom I had no direct control. I also had to command and lead each of my subordinate organizations, ensuring they understood the vision associated with the conduct of kinetic (combat) and nonkinetic (noncombat engagement) operations within their vastly different battle spaces. I had to communicate with all those in the task force and all those who supported or reported on the actions of the task force, including senior military leaders, congressional visitors (who were in effect my "bosses"), as well as a bevy of family members and media representatives. I also had to continue leading those around me: my staff, my subordinate commanders, and the team that traveled with me.

Every leader needs to keep a finger on the pulse of what's happening within his or her organization, and in my case, that meant I needed to get a daily feel for how our soldiers engaged both the enemy and our Iraqi friends. And so each day, I flew from our headquarters in Tikrit to a forward operating base or combat outpost to do a battlefield circulation.

Besides the two pilots and the two crew chiefs who managed the Black Hawk helicopter that flew us to our daily destination, we always had a relatively small party of young NCOs and my aide-de-camp. The noncommissioned officers served in my personal security detail, tasked with ensuring the US would not suffer the embarrassment of getting an American general killed in combat. Finally, the group included my communication sergeant, responsible to make certain I could talk to anyone, from anywhere, with a satellite hookup.

Sergeant Smith, whom we all called "Smitty," was the best "commo" sergeant in the business. Short and muscular, he always had a smile tugging at his lips, as though he'd just thought of a joke but couldn't quite decide if it would be appropriate to pass on to a general. Whenever I pressed him to tell me his thoughts, he always responded. But he never crossed the line of the appropriate senior/subordinate relationship, though occasionally he came pretty close. His best trait was how he combined his straight talk with humor.

One day, we made the forty-five-minute flight from Tikrit to Mosul to conduct a battlefield circulation with a group from the US Third Armored Cavalry Regiment and also an element from the Second Iraqi Infantry Division. On the flight we discussed leadership. I enjoyed engaging with young soldiers as they started to form their own leadership philosophies. Our conversation over the helicopter's intercom made us forget, at least for the moment, the intense heat and the perils of the mission in front of us. Smitty seemed particularly interested in the topic of a leader's "bearing" or "presence."

"Sir," he asked over the intercom, "what do you think is the best way to show presence? There's only one of you and yet there are thousands in this task force. How do you make others aware of your 'presence' or 'bearing' when you're in charge of something as big as Task Force Iron?"

"Smitty," I answered, "the most important thing I've ever learned about bearing and presence in leadership is something I heard from General Dempsey: Whenever you're in charge of others, leaders don't have the right to have a bad day.

"Leaders are always on stage, providing an example and portraying that it's always a great day. Leaders can never look upset or annoyed or about to blow—unless, of course, they want to look that way for effect. The reason for always being upbeat is that any organization, even a big one, takes on the personality of the leader. And when you're a leader, someone is always looking. If you're grumpy, the organization will wonder what's wrong with you—and then worse, they'll start exhibiting that grumpiness."

Marty Dempsey is a dear friend who had been my boss when he commanded the First Armored Division in Baghdad from 2003–4. He told his subordinates that when they found themselves under the toughest situations, they had to remain upbeat, even if everything seemed to be going wrong. Leaders had to remain calm and above the fray. If leaders demonstrated this positive example, the entire organization, even an entire army, was more likely to maintain a winning attitude. But as soon as a leader became sour or seemed defeated, the organization would soon follow. General Dempsey, of course, went on to receive four stars and become the chairman of the Joint Chiefs of Staff and the senior military advisor to the president.

When we arrived at Mosul, we promised each other we would continue our leadership discussion another day. After disembarking, we found ourselves walking the labyrinthine streets of the Mosul market. Parts of this market might be considered "unappetizing," especially the open sewers, ditches with all sorts of unmentionable green stuff floating among feces and mud. The foul smells matched some of the sights. On the positive side, however, we felt relieved to see a thriving economy and a relatively friendly population. We exchanged multiple greetings of as-saalam alakum and as-salaam with Iraqi shopkeepers. They smiled and returned the Arabic greeting.

A good sign, I thought.

As we left the market area to return to the FOB, however, we came under sniper fire from the rooftops of some high-rise buildings. Reacting to contact, we immediately assumed firing positions in the only cover available, the ditches filled with green and brown sludge. With Smitty on one side and one of my security men on the other, all of us quickly got covered with the muddy, stinking sewage.

A groan and complaint almost left my lips when Smitty stopped me before I could say a word. With a big smile, he leaned over and whispered, "Hey, sir, it's a great (censored) day, isn't it?"

I could only smile back. My earlier leadership lesson, so easy to rattle off in the relatively safe, antiseptic environment of the back of a Black Hawk helicopter, had just intersected the real world of Mosul and combat. Smitty was now leading me in what I would call a "leading-up" approach, reminding me I had to walk the walk as much as I talked the talk. He nudged me to be that positive leader in not-so-great times. Unlike me, Smitty had managed to keep a smile, even as we all found each other in that reeking ditch. I deeply appreciated his reminder of my own near-failure of leadership and the way he quickly got me back on track.

CHAPTER 5

The Art of Leading Up

Michael Useem's book, *Leading Up: How to Lead Your Boss So You Both Win*, describes a variety of situations in which several leaders faced some difficult challenges. All leaders, he says, at times need to nudge their bosses to do something that will result in organizational success. Since some do this well and others don't, some succeed while others fail.

Useem tells one story in which a governmental leader attempted to present a future opportunity for a trade agreement with China—but his boss couldn't imagine it. Another story details a failed ascent of Mount Everest that resulted in multiple deaths, mainly because the expedition's leaders wouldn't listen to their guides, and the guides didn't know how to lead up.

Many of Useem's anecdotes describe military relationships, one with General Lee and President Jefferson Davis during the Civil War, another with General Peter Pace and all of his bosses in Southern Command. Useem explains how the factors associated with "leading up" either contributed to or obstructed mission success.

In any high-performing organization, a leader who wants to truly help a superior to accomplish a worthy mission has a responsibility to furnish the boss with candid and transparent insight, advice, and options. That's called "leading up" and it's also dyadic, "one-on-one." The same leadership techniques that apply to subordinates and peers can be adjusted to interact with superiors.

Slip into the Boss's Shoes

In every case where a leader has to "lead up," it's important to remember that superiors often have a much more complex view of the terrain and strategic implications of the situation. That makes it incumbent upon subordinate leaders to understand the leader's intent and the implications of the situation.

While it's easier to say, "The boss just doesn't get it," proper leading up entails not only an understanding of the boss's personal motivation, but also the relative importance of any particular issue that may compete in the boss's list of priorities. To lead up, then, subordinate leaders must place themselves in the bosses' shoes and try to understand motivation from a more strategic perspective.

In every situation that Useem describes in his book, for example, the leader attempting to "lead up" possessed:

- *Strong and obvious personal values; each leader held values that positively contributed to her life's purpose.*

- *A desire to help the organization achieve a goal, whether linked to winning a war, reaching a mountaintop, or building a successful business venture.*

- *The ability to lead their organization; unfortunately, several of the leaders could not apply the same techniques when influencing their bosses, which resulted in failure to meet the stated objective.*

- *True humility and a desire to learn (in those scenarios that resulted in success). In every situation that resulted in failure, the leader exhibited an abundance of pride or hubris, which negatively affected his relationship with the boss. That, in turn, contributed to mission failure.*

- *A strong communication ability; those who succeeded knew how to speak to power, while those who failed never understood a superior's motivation.*

- *The element of respect and the ability to generate trust, obvious in every successful situation but missing in the failed operations.*

Regardless of how challenging the situation might seem, applying the fundamentals of leadership can have a profound effect. The movie *Saving Private Ryan* has some good illustrations in this regard.

The film portrayed what happened after General George Marshall made a decision to find and safely bring home the remaining son of Mrs. Ryan, after her three other sons died in combat. It also depicted the uniquely different perspective of a group of soldiers led by Captain Miller (brilliantly played by Tom Hanks), who griped about putting their lives on the line for a mission they didn't understand.

Captain Miller deftly described to his men how the dangers the squad faced fit into the grander scale. Not only did Captain Miller describe to his soldiers what was going on at the strategic level, in language they could understand, but he also exhibited great leadership traits in not being negatively affected by his soldiers' emotional reactions to the dangerous task at hand. Additionally, he provided insights into his personal values and why he saw the accomplishment of the mission—saving Private Ryan—as extremely important.

Jay's Real-Life Example

When I think of the finer points of leading up, I think of the real-life experiences of Colonel (retired) Jay Voorhees, who worked under my command in the Twelfth Combat Aviation Brigade in Europe.

Jay had spent most of his career with Special Operations Aviation units, which support what we call "unconventional" forces. Jay had commanded pilots and their helicopters in some of the most intense and secret operations of the Iraq and Afghan wars. When he reached the rank of colonel, the army selected him to command its largest aviation brigade, the Twelfth, a unit with more than one hundred helicopters and five thousand soldiers. But he'd have to operate in Europe, a theater where he had never served.

Jay became one of my subordinate brigade commanders on the eve of the unit deploying for a twelve-month combat tour to Afghanistan. Because we had never met, he knew he needed to quickly prove to me his competence and his leadership abilities. As a new and unknown commander heading into combat, he needed to quickly earn my trust.

Jay developed a plan to lead his organization and influence me. He talked to a variety of people to learn more about me. Already he had gained all sorts of intelligence about his command: their assigned tasks, their training calendar to prepare for deployment, the personality of his subordinates, and their skills and achievements. He also recognized the importance of scouting out his new commanding general. He needed to know my likes, my dislikes, my hot buttons, and the agenda I had set for the entire organization.

At the time, US Army Europe numbered more than twenty brigades and sixty thousand soldiers. Jay understood that while his organization was important to me, it also was just one of the many units that needed my attention. He also took the time to learn from others how I operated. When I visited units, for example, I had a certain set of expectations for meeting people, discussing maintenance and training, spending time with soldiers and their families, doing physical training, and eating in the chow hall with troops and younger leaders. Most importantly, I had a certain disdain for long PowerPoint presentations. He anticipated that I would likely visit his unit within thirty days of him taking command, and he wanted to be ready.

As a dedicated professional, Jay conducted a lot of preliminary analysis focused on understanding problems, his new environment, and the personality and motivations of his superior. He talked to a lot of people who already had a handle on these things. His actions as a new commander set the stage for making a good first impression, and they also showed the importance of establishing trust within an organization. His hard work paid off in how his unit came to be viewed, how his ideas were accepted, and how his organization achieved its objectives, in both Europe and Afghanistan.

All of this resulted from Jay "leading up." He understood motivation, used selfless influence techniques, communicated effectively, and established obtainable standards and objectives. When Jay felt the crush of combat on several tough missions, the trust he had built with me contributed to a better understanding and more effective mission accomplishment.

Leading Up in Healthcare

During the PLD seminar on "leading up," we reframed some techniques of how to lead and applied them to engagements with those in the organization's hierarchy. Many participants seemed eager to give the ideas a try, mainly because they wanted to get their bosses to do what they wanted them to do.

But we turned the tables on our participants. Instead of asking them to investigate how open their bosses appeared to be to new ideas, we asked them to report how *they* reacted when their own subordinates wanted to present ideas that challenged their usual processes and systems. We gave them only one task: "Talk to one subordinate, one peer, and one supervisor, and ask them this question: 'What are some things I do that make it a challenge for you to deal with me? And please give me some suggestions on how I can improve in my interactions.'"

Most of our physicians had never been asked to request candid feedback on their interpersonal skills. Their reports, however, made it clear they had acquired new insights that would help them in their leadership journey. One physician received some especially harsh feedback from an office manager and a resident. He told the group, "This assignment was a lot harder than I thought it would be." And what made it so difficult? He cited several issues:

> First, I had never asked for feedback, so it was hard for me to ask the question.
>
> Second, and just as interesting, it didn't appear any of the people I approached had ever been put on the spot that way. I queried two people: my office manager and one of my senior residents. After initially dodging the question, my resident finally provided a torrent of responses.
>
> She said I procrastinate on issues I know might result in conflict. She then said I'm a great boss, but I choose to focus on short-term goals while failing to provide a long-term vision for the practice. We're growing, and everyone is happy with that, but she told me no one really knows where we're going.
>
> Then she hesitated and said I'm too busy all the time... that I'm too nice of a guy, and that I sometimes allow people to take advantage of me. She said I should expect more from her and from the rest of my staff; they are all willing to do more, but they view me as wanting to do everything myself.
>
> Then she said something I never thought I would hear,

since we have such a great team: that everyone loves working for me, but sometimes it appears I don't trust them.

I really learned a lot from that discussion, and I was really glad she was so honest with me.

Next, a surgical specialist reported on his interaction with the head of the emergency department at his hospital:

> I talked to the ER doc, who I like a lot and who I work with a lot. I asked, "What can I do better in communicating with you?"
>
> He didn't delay a nanosecond. He immediately looked me in the eye and said, "You multitask too much." He said I was always reading my phone when others were talking to me, sometimes even patients and their families. And then he said, "Most times, when I'm telling you the history of a patient, you're not listening to me. You take the chart, start flipping through it, and it's obvious you're not paying attention to the things I'm reporting that we've learned in the ED. You immediately jump to the diagnosis, which makes me feel you're not listening to me or how I can contribute to the care of the patient. I'm concerned someday you're really going to miss something important."
>
> He even told me he had mentioned this to me once before, but I responded that I was going to see the patient and that I like to get the story directly from him.
>
> I really thought I had good communication with this doctor, but it is apparent he doesn't see it the same way. I learned a big lesson from this: I have to look people in the eye, be quiet, listen actively, and really see things from the other person's perspective before doing what I think I need to do.

Finally, we heard from an outspoken and good-natured doctor who had been appointed as a director just after the PLD course began. He was in the early stages of "formal" leadership:

> I asked four people to give me feedback: One is an AdventHealth vice president who oversees a service line with which I interact; another is a nurse practitioner with whom I work very closely every day; a third is my unit nurse manager; and the last is a charge nurse. I tried to pick people I thought would be honest with me, but initially I received compliment, compliment, compliment, "You're the best guy ever," compliment, compliment, "You're a pleasure to work with," "You're a truly remarkable teacher," "You're an exceptional leader," blah, blah, blah.
>
> Then I asked them to type things up and give me anonymous feedback, instead of talking directly to me. I reminded them I really needed to get some honest criticism, or Mark and Jay wouldn't believe I had anything to report! Here are some quotes from those anonymous notes:
>
> • *You can sometimes be judgmental with those you find less competent.*
>
> • *The weaker members of the nursing staff find it hard to approach you.*
>
> • *You're always right with your medical assessments, but sometimes you can be a jerk in showing off about it.*
>
> • *You set a high standard for yourself for clinical practice, and you go about achieving it through hard work and discipline. You expect the same high standards from everyone you work with,*

but you usually don't tell them what your standards are or what you're looking for, so people are confused.

- *People like you, but they also want to contribute to the team. Delegate more!*

These comments really made me think. I know I have high expectations, but I now realize I was assuming everyone in the practice had the same level of expertise and understanding I have... but they don't. I've concluded that I need to be more humble, more interactive, more in the teaching mode. I should reach out more, counsel, and coach.

The best "leading up" starts with making sure that others can "lead up" to you! Leaders who lack the humility or wisdom to listen to the perspectives of their subordinates seldom have a lot of success leading up to their own superiors. What goes around comes around, I guess, and that applies in both a positive and a negative direction.

Can We Talk?

Mike, one of our PLD physicians, said to me one day, "Can we talk? I've got a problem, and I'm hoping to get some advice and perhaps some help."

Mike explained that he and his superior weren't seeing eye-to-eye on a particular issue. The doctor felt disheartened, not knowing how he should address the problem and how he might generate some trust with his boss.

"We just discussed this kind of situation a few weeks ago," I said. "Are you seeing this as an opportunity to 'lead up'?"

Mike said he'd thought of that, which is why he'd come by. But he suspected he needed a bit more instruction on the kind of analysis and the type of approach he should take in talking to others about his boss's likes, dislikes, and agenda items.

"Oh, I get it," I said. "You want *me* to help you get into his inner circle, gain his trust, and repair this bad blood."

He smiled sheepishly. "You got it," he answered.

Since Mike had internalized one of the important elements of leading up—reaching out to others for help in understanding the motivations and personality of a superior—I contacted another administrator and we independently approached his boss to discuss the situation. Those conversations opened the door for an improved relationship between Mike and his boss. While the pair didn't become best friends, they did manage to smooth out their interactions, which led to a big win for the organization.

And isn't that what leadership is all about?

QUESTIONS FOR REFLECTION AND DISCUSSION

1. What motivates your boss, and what are his/her top three priorities? How are you contributing to helping achieve those priorities?

2. What things do you do that make it a challenge for subordinates to work with you?

3. How easy is it to communicate with your boss? Does he listen intently, or do you have challenges in getting your point across? How would your team or your patient answer this question in talking about you?

WAR STORY

When You Start to Feel Overwhelmed

So there we were...

In the spring of 2007, my boss—a four-star general and the
commander of all army forces in Europe—arrived unexpectedly at
my office, closed the door, and congratulated me on being selected
as the next commander of the First Armored Division. The news both
shocked and honored me. Shocked, because I never thought I would be
named to command one of the ten army divisions. Honored, because
"First Tank" was the army's only named armored division, a unit I had
served with in combat twice before. I knew that about twenty or so
other two-star generals also coveted this command of eighteen thousand
soldiers in a storied organization.

The general told me I would take command in about a month. That
was the easy and fun part. The harder and more challenging part was
hearing I would have to prepare the headquarters of the division, about
one thousand soldiers, for an unexpected and unplanned deployment
to Iraq as part of the "surge." My boss also informed me that the other

seventeen thousand soldiers of the division would not accompany me, as they would be deployed to other missions and units as part of the European drawdown.

I would have to build what the army termed a "modular task force" comprised of units from a variety of locations in a process many in the Pentagon had called a "plug-in and play" arrangement. While the tactic had been tried on a smaller scale, the European-based First Armored would be the first division ever to go to war with a variety of other organizations. I would command units and go into combat with those who had not trained with me, working with subordinate commanders I had never met.

A ground combat brigade has between four and seven thousand soldiers, based on its designation as infantry, armored, air assault, Stryker, airborne, or cavalry. Each unit type comes from a different "tribe" and culture. I began the deployment with a Stryker brigade from Louisiana, an infantry brigade from upstate New York, an armored brigade from Texas, and an air assault brigade from Kentucky. Over the course of our fifteen-month tour, those units would get replaced with a cavalry brigade from a post in Texas and then another armored brigade from the same state, a Stryker brigade from Hawaii, and then another Stryker brigade from Alaska. The helicopters associated with a three thousand-plus soldier aviation brigade would come from Kansas, the engineers from Missouri, and the artillery from Oklahoma. Our military police battalion would join us from Hawaii while our explosive ordinance teams and civil affairs units would come from reserve and National Guard units representing twenty-seven states.

Additionally, our task force would include elements from the US Navy and US Air Force, and I also would have responsibility for coalition forces from Poland, Georgia, Lithuania, and Korea. Part of the mission required us to coordinate the recruitment, training, and employment of four newly formed Iraqi army divisions (about sixty-five thousand soldiers total) and province police forces (about forty thousand policemen). The cherries on top were the valued members of the US State Department, along with various governmental and nongovernmental agencies that worked in our area. I had to ensure the care, safety, and successful mission conduct of all these individuals and organizations.

Clearly, my ability to use character, presence, and intellect to lead, develop, and achieve results would get tested in this new mission. My competencies to understand motivation, use various measures of influence, communicate vision, and accomplish organizational objectives would get severely challenged in this job. I would have plenty of opportunities to engage in myriad dyadic interchanges with a variety of individuals boasting various ranks and coming from an assortment of dissimilar cultures.

But now the job requirement would extend beyond one-on-one leadership engagements. New demands would center on forming and enriching this vast new team. I had to help everyone understand how to share ownership of the objectives I would receive from my superior. We needed to defeat a complex insurgency, build a stronger Iraqi security force, contribute to the stability of the Iraqi people, and improve the functioning of the provincial and regional governments in Northern Iraq.

I immediately went into high gear with a small cell to analyze the Iraq mission and determine how best to prepare in the short time that remained before deploying. At our home station in Wiesbaden, Germany, we designed the actions that Task Force Iron would undertake in both the short and the long term after arriving in Iraq. We discussed ways to prepare for the personalities and culture of the various groups that would soon join our team. Forming that team would be my greatest challenge. I knew I would have to build trust, communicate expectations, develop metrics to measure success, receive feedback from individuals I had never worked with, influence people beyond their comfort zone, and accomplish seemingly impossible tasks. To do all those things, you need to know your organization well—but you also need to deeply understand the challenges your organization faces.

One critically important part of the plan focused on how I would meet all the new commanders and their organizations in the shortest possible period of time, given that combat operations could not wait. I established a goal of getting to more than fifty locations and spending time with more than one hundred commanders and their units in the first ninety days, all while executing the tasks that only I could accomplish.

My best friend, my wife, could sense I felt overwhelmed with all of this. When I returned home late one night, she handed me two quotes on a small piece of paper. The first came from an anonymous source:

> When faced with a monumental challenge, mere mortals often shiver in the shadow of its immensity. Mere mortals look up and think they will never be able to scale the heights. But leaders know any mountain can be conquered one toehold at a time; they know it is the rock face in front of them that needs their undivided attention if they want to make it to the top. The leader doesn't look up in despair or look down in fear, he just climbs.

The second note, less philosophic, featured the words of the actor/entertainer Will Smith: "I do not have to build a perfect wall today. I just have to lay one perfect brick."

Sue suspected these quotes would help me better understand that any leader can accomplish any difficult task involving a large and complex organization if he or she focuses on building a team, generating trust, and tackling the tasks, one task at a time. She urged me to focus on the fundamentals, use the strengths of my experiences and the team, and to apply all available resources. But she also reminded me that success in climbing a mountain or building a perfect wall comes slowly.

In all my experiences before receiving this most challenging combat assignment, I had learned several things that I would apply to the upcoming mission. But in handing me these notes, Sue taught me one more important lesson. While I could take comfort from the advice written on the paper, I also realized that anyone attempting a grand mission with a large organization had better have at least one best friend to provide feedback and encouragement.

CHAPTER 6

Building Trust in Different Kinds of Teams

E arly in my army career, I learned a simple truth. While politicians and high-ranking government officials may believe "the national interest" or a "solid security strategy" or a high-minded "military mission" might be the reason soldiers fight and accomplish extraordinarily difficult tasks, in fact, those things don't feel terribly important to soldiers at the pointed end of a spear. While a military team might find the objectives of the nation helpful in understanding *what* they are being asked to do, the reason *why* soldiers go into harm's way is much easier to understand.

The simple truth is that soldiers in good organizations do seemingly impossible things because they do not want to let down their immediate leaders and fellow soldiers. They do not want to fail, *because they do not want their team to fail.*

The army uses seven key characteristics to define effective teams. For an army team to succeed, soldiers must operate in an environment of trust, whether trust in their leaders or trust in their fellow soldiers. Soldiers must know the standards each member of the team is required to meet, and each soldier must know he or she will be held accountable to meet those standards. Soldiers must also be assured that every other team member will be held accountable for meeting them. Like any athletic team preparing for a competition, soldiers must have confidence in their own abilities as well as in the abilities of their leaders and the other members of their team. While missions vary, each soldier knows he or she will be asked to contribute in a specific way to meet or exceed specific challenges to get the job done. And after accomplishing the mission, soldiers expect to be rewarded for their individual and team accomplishments.

Could the same be said of most healthcare teams?

What Strong Teams Have in Common

What are the defining features of a successful healthcare organization? Knowing these characteristics will help physician leaders understand what strong teams have in common in the operating room, in a practice or group, on the hospital's medical staff, or on any other team.

What are some effective techniques associated with leading organizations in different stages of formation or development? Understanding this is important for doctors asked to form and lead new teams, or if they get placed in existing formal positions with the requirement to find new solutions to old problems.

We'll look at all of that in a moment, but first, perhaps, we should stop and ask ourselves what we mean by "team." A team is more than a group that comes together to "do something." A team has some common purpose. But how is that purpose communicated? Who in the group has the job of coordinating the effort? Who defines the limits of "doing something," and who ensures that "something" gets accomplished on time and to standard? Which member of the group will pull the rest together in a unifying purpose and ensure it stays together until the job is done? What kind of individuals should be recruited to the group, and who should be excused because he or she fails to contribute to the successful accomplishment of the task? A group, in and of itself, does not necessarily constitute a team.

Words are powerful. Mark Twain once said that using the right word at the right time, in the right way, is the difference between the lightning bug and the lightning.

I contend that to properly lead any team, it's important first to define the word. Here's one definition:

> A team is a group of people linked in common purpose that is required to execute tasks high in complexity, or tasks that may have multiple independent subtasks which would be difficult to accomplish outside the dynamics of the group.

Team members have complementary knowledge and skills. Teams generate synergy and achieve success through coordinated efforts. Finding or growing the right people who evolve into a team is the first step in gaining smooth efficiency, true effectiveness, and high standards.

And *all* of that requires a leader with highly developed leadership skills.

Leaders must recruit the right people to be part of the team, and then they must train and drill those teammates to meet norms and standards established by the leader. The leader must provide a clear vision to chart a direction for the members of the team, providing the boundaries for "open-field running" and keeping them in line if they start to stray or underperform. The team leader also must remain singularly focused, like a laser, to provide the will, the energy, and the drive for those on the team to accomplish the task.

Depending on the personality and strengths or weaknesses of any given leader, teams can perform miracles, fail miserably, or achieve some limited success. But it is the leader who makes it all happen, for good or for ill.

Characteristics of a Successful Team

Think for a moment about the seven key words I used at the beginning of this chapter to define effective teams:

- *Trust*
- *Standards*
- *Accountability*
- *Confidence*

- *Teamwork*
- *Challenge*
- *Rewards*

These seven words represent hard work, dedication to the members of the team, allocation of time and resources, tough decisions, and applied interpersonal skills on the part of a leader. I know of no mnemonic, memory trick, or acronym that helps leaders remember these seven words. But I have found each of them is critically important to building and leading teams.

As a commander at many levels in the military, I've unfortunately had to conduct investigations as to why some units failed to accomplish their missions. At several of our army's training centers, I've also had to tell subordinate unit commanders they could not deploy their units until they fixed some glaring problem, because that issue might get someone killed or prevent the success of the mission. On every occasion, the explanatory report might include phrases like "failure to adhere to established standards" or "lack of trust in established processes that prevented the proper execution of the mission" or "the members of the team did not have confidence in the ability of their unit to accomplish the task." But no matter what ended up in the formal report and no matter the discrepancies observed in a deployment rehearsal, the inadequacy of any team to accomplish a mission *always* boiled down to leaders who failed to adhere to the ideas summed up in those seven critical words.

Good leaders understand the crucial implications of those seven words. They recognize that the words apply to every team situation, including teams in healthcare. These become part of the leader's *competencies* of leading-developing-achieving (introduced in Chapter 3).

- *Teams must trust their leaders to do the right things, for the right reasons. The leader's character, presence, and intellect must contribute to the atmosphere of trust that helps the team function effectively. The leader must be the driving force in building trust with each individual and with the team as a whole.*

- *Teams must know the standards of care, team members' individual responsibilities, and the ways in which each member is expected to interact. Team members must know they will be held accountable by other members of the team and their leader if they cannot execute their skills or if they cannot contribute effectively. The leader outlines the required standards; the leader is responsible for ensuring all team members know their roles and how they are expected to contribute as a member of the team.*

- *Each team member must have confidence in his or her own skills, whether that team member is the attending nurse, the radiologist, the transporter, the receptionist, or the doctor. Each team member must feel confident that the other members of the team know their skills and can synchronize their action as part of the team when asked to serve a patient, treat an injury, save a life, or solve a problem. The leader is responsible for forming the team and ensuring the competencies of every member and the group as a whole; the leader is responsible for taking action to correct any team shortcomings.*

- *The team must be challenged to grow, both as individuals and as a collective, in competence, confidence, and team skills. Each member of the team must continuously evolve according to the demands of an ever-changing healthcare environment; doing so will allow the team to increasingly provide the best care possible. Leaders enforce and reinforce this growth requirement, and leaders challenge the team members and the entire team to understand their responsibility for professional and personal growth.*

- *Teams must receive recognition—praise, promotion, advancement, or money—which will help reinforce contributions to the team and to the organization. Leaders are responsible for appropriately recognizing members of their team.*

Great leadership makes all these things happen. These are the competencies of great leaders. Leaders establish the element of trust in the team, they determine individual and team standards, and then they relentlessly hold the team accountable for attaining those standards. Leaders develop confidence, in each individual and in the team as a whole, by making available opportunities for personal and professional growth. Leaders find every effort to build upon individual and team confidence through an insistence on teamwork. Effective leaders challenge their organization by outlining achievable goals. And leaders reward key contributions and team efforts.

If you think, *Wait a minute! Aren't these the responsibilities of the CEO or the hospital administrator?* No doubt. Most, but certainly not all, executives inherently understand and apply these elements in their organization. But to be a successful leader at any level, whether on a small three-person team or a large, global corporation, an understanding of the implications of each of these seven words contributes significantly to mission accomplishment. Physicians who want to be great leaders must apply these approaches to their team and then practice leading at every level.

The point is that all good leaders do all of these things with any team, big or small. Physicians who want to become known as leaders must recognize these requirements and, depending on the situation, apply each of the criteria with varying degrees to patients, with other healthcare teammates in day-to-day situations, or when they achieve some formal position in the executive hierarchy.

Leader Responsibilities in Building Successful Teams

Let's take a more detailed look at each of the responsibilities any leader must embrace and the competencies they must exhibit to build successful teams.

Trust

The leader must be the driving force in building trust with each member of the team and with the team as a whole. Every team member should believe in the words and actions of the leader. The key leader *attributes* listed under the categories of *character-presence-intellect* all contribute to building trust. Before accomplishing any objective, team members will want to feel sure the team leader is considering the organization's goals. They also will want to know their leader is keeping the well-being of team members at the forefront. The leader's words and actions must remain in sync so that what the leader believes plays out in what he or she does. Any deviation can contribute to a loss of trust, and trust is the most critical element of successful leadership. Strong trust between the leader and the led means all things are achievable.

Trust is critically important in the relationship between doctor and patient. When patients perceive that the physician seems focused on their well-being, rather than on the fee charged or the number of patients in the waiting room, trust grows. When the physician spends time explaining a procedure while sitting next to a patient in a hospital room, the patient will have more confidence in the healthcare team. Multiple studies have shown that when a doctor sits down in a patient's room to explain a procedure or talk about a prognosis, that simple act of sitting significantly improves "physician communication" scores on the HCAHPS. In one study, a physician stood in one room for the same amount of time he sat in another room, while communicating information to two different patients. Patients who observed the doctor seated for their appointment consistently believed that the physician visited for a longer period of time.[14]

Equally important, physician leaders who want to lead healthcare organizations must develop the same kind of trust with executives. Gaining a reputation for teamwork, showing a desire to improve healthcare, engaging to overcome misunderstanding, and building consensus will all contribute to a physician's success in dealing with healthcare administrators.

Just before operation Desert Storm began, General Fred Franks, the commander of the 140,000-soldier VII Corps, visited a unit on the front lines. He launched into a long-winded explanation of the corps' battle plan with a team of soldiers from a tank platoon. After he finished, one young soldier stepped forward and said: "Don't worry, General, we trust you. We know you've thought this through and you're going to do everything you can to win this fight and bring us back home. Sir, we trust you. We don't have to know everything you've planned, just like you don't need to know everything we've done to get ready. But we trust you, and you can trust us to get it done at our level."

Standards and Accountability

The leader must outline the required standards and ensure all team members understand their roles and know that they will be held accountable as members of the team. Leaders must therefore know the standards and enforce them. If the standards have become outdated or inappropriate, it is the leader's responsibility to change them through an approved process. Leaders who ensure adherence to standards through teaching, coaching, counseling, and mentoring are critically important to achieving any objective. A leader's adherence to standards is also important as an example in establishing trust in his or her leadership.

For this reason, we insisted that each PLD class begin precisely at noon. Before we launched the class, many administrators who worked regularly with physicians warned us that we'd be lucky to get all the participants to every class. They also predicted that many physicians would show up late. Since such a standard was unacceptable to us, we established a new standard at the first seminar: "Since all of you were fortunate enough to be selected to attend this course, we expect you to show up on time, prepared for every class." We insisted that participants be seated at the designated start time... and we locked the door to ensure compliance.

We believed that if participants rightfully expected their instructors to be punctual and prepared, then we had an equally valid expectation that they show the same courtesy and respect to us. Early on, some class participants thought of this insistence as an example of our quirky military background. But once we communicated this standard and enforced it on one occasion, we had few incidents of tardiness. Establishing guidelines for punctuality and preparation became a standard for the course; it also became a vehicle for generating trust. If seminar members arrived on time, then they could trust their instructors to present five hours' worth of leadership learning.

But we also had a nuanced teaching point. If our PLD physicians eventually got placed in a formal leadership role and the CEO called them to an important meeting, then they had better be on time. When a leader comes late to a meeting with the boss, that tardiness *will* tarnish their professional reputation. One of the most important things about being a leader is showing up on time. Interestingly, our corporate CEO was interested in the Physician Leader Course, and asked if I would set up a meeting with him and any "volunteer" doctors. I asked the class, and twenty-three of our doctors said they would enjoy conversing with him. I gave them no guidance and was surprised when the CEO called me the next day. He enjoyed the engagement, but then made a point of telling me that every single physician was waiting outside his office ten minutes before the scheduled meeting. He mentioned that was the first time he had ever held a meeting where at least one doctor didn't show up late!

Physician leaders at any level of an organization are required to set standards. In every area—such as how a staff runs a private practice, the way a surgical team communicates during a robotic surgery, or making recommendations for new approaches in an evolving healthcare profession—physician leaders have to set the standards. Some need to be written, some can be passed from employee-to-employee or from physician-to-executive, but all need to be enforced to make for an efficient and effective organization. This is required for proper teaching, coaching, and counseling, and this leadership skill is applicable whether working with a small team or a large healthcare organization.

"A great leader never walks by a standards violation," a great non-commissioned officer once told me. "If you walk past it and you don't correct it, then you've just established a new, lower standard."

Leaders are also required to *coach* their teams as to the leader's expectations of achieving standards and to *counsel* their teams regarding accountability in meeting those standards.

Coaching means helping someone understand, and then perform, a task. A coach helps team members understand their current level of performance and instructs them on how to reach the next level. Coaches understand how the task best contributes to the effectiveness of the organization. Those getting coached may need work on learning a skill or perfecting a skill, but the coach will help them understand their current level of performance while giving them instruction on how to improve, contribute to the team, and to reach the next level.

Coaching is usually one-way: "Here's what you're doing, here's what I'd like you to do instead, so you and everyone around you can perform at peak effectiveness. Here's what you need to do to make that happen." This technique can be applied to someone in a new position, as well as to someone who is learning unfamiliar skills or adjusting from old ones. When a leader is "leading up" and attempting to "coach" a superior, more nuance is required in describing what that individual is doing and how he or she can better contribute. For example: "Hey boss, I really liked the way you communicated that requirement, but some of us might better understand what you want us to do if you…"

Leaders use the process of counseling to review another individual's performance and explain how that performance contributes to the potential of the organization. It is always interactive. Both the leader and the led—whether a subordinate, a peer, or a superior—are active participants in a two-way discussion geared toward identifying strengths and weaknesses in individual and organizational performance.

Many nurses and administrators have received counseling as part of executive performance reports. Clinicians at AdventHealth Orlando actively participate in "H-S-L Counseling." H-S-L stands for High-Solid-Low, where various aspects of the nurses' skill sets are placed in one of those categories for quarterly counseling sessions. Those who receive marks consistently in the "High" category are given new challenges, promoted to advanced positions, and rewarded with pay raises. Those in the "Solid" are told how they can improve; their raters give them input as to performance objectives and timelines for accomplishing advanced tasks. Those who receive marks in the "Low" category receive extensive counseling and coaching to improve their performance; if they do not improve, they are terminated from employment after a prescribed period.

Physicians, however, almost never receive formal performance counseling.

Inexperienced leaders nearly always feel uncomfortable with both coaching and counseling, but physician leaders need to understand how their roles in these helpful activities can translate to upholding and polishing adherence to standards, establishing team accountability, and forming high-performance organizations. Most people *want* feedback on their performance, especially feedback given in an empathetic and positive way. High standards and positive feedback are crucial elements of good leadership.

Confidence and Teamwork

The leader is responsible to ensure the competencies of every member of the team and for the team as a whole. And it is the leader's responsibility to take action to correct any shortcomings.

A candid discussion of skills can define future performance objectives and contribute to an individual's confidence in his or her ability to contribute to the team. When combined with various coaching techniques, such as defining the individual's strengths and developmental needs with an eye toward achieving improvement, or finding ways to eliminate developmental barriers that hinder improved performance, these skills are critical to leading individuals.

Healthcare leaders are familiar with M&M (mortality and morbidity) reviews. These events analyze and reconstruct some procedure that resulted in an unfavorable outcome. Lessons learned from these reviews normally contribute to better patient treatment.

AdventHealth Orlando requires an increased use of "Physician-Nurse Rounding," in which nurses are expected to "round" at certain time intervals, address specific issues with every patient during each round, and keep records of the conduct of the event, records that could be inspected by the chief clinical officer or chief medical officer. Doctors are required to accompany nurses on select rounds and must comply with specific requirements for exchanging information about each patient on the ward. While rounding is certainly not a new technique, ensuring a rigorous time schedule and conducting specific checks is contributing to an improved perception of better healthcare by patients.

Along the same lines, several of our PLD physicians participated in a newly launched training regimen called "Physician Shadowing." In this program, physicians are "shadowed" by others who use a checklist to evaluate various aspects of physician engagement and communication, bedside manner, transfer of information, and physician-nurse interaction. The evaluator then provides a critique on specific areas after observing the interactions between doctors, nurses, other members of the healthcare team, and patients and their families.

While programs like Physician-Nurse Rounding and Physician Shadowing might contribute to improved physician leadership, improved communication and better patient interaction can certainly show health-care leaders practical ways to improve their effectiveness.

The army's method of conducting AAR (After-Action Review) might also prove useful to help healthcare organizations improve their teams, develop their coaching and counseling techniques, and improve their leadership skills. Every AAR is facilitated by a disinterested party who wants to help the leader improve the organization, no matter the size or mission of the team. The facilitator, an expert in whatever he or she is asked to observe, witnesses an event in which the team has focused on achieving some specific result. While observing the event, the facilitator makes note of what transpires, why it likely occurred, and which members of the team contributed to positive or negative outcomes. In more robust AARs, the facilitator uses cameras or audio devices that provide inarguable "ground truth" for the observation, and the audio or video may be presented during the review.

AARs are either chronological reviews of activities or are more tightly focused on a few key issues selected by the team leader to determine how to improve outcomes. After reviewing the actions, the leader takes responsibility for establishing new standards, reinforcing accountabilities, changing responsibilities, or improving training designed to improve skills that contribute to individual proficiency or collective competency. The review allows participation by all members, so even the leader may learn how to improve his or her performance. At the end of the AAR, the leader is required to assign responsibility for who will affect the change and the timeline for the fixes to take place. The result is always improved individual confidence and better teamwork.

Challenge

Leaders enforce the requirement for each team member and the entire team to grow professionally and personally. A variety of approaches are used to challenge individuals and teams, important for both individual and group self-actualization. A leader can prescribe personal or team performance targets (generated during the coaching, counseling, or AAR process), or set goals in conjunction with members of the team. The leader must take care in assigning goals, as it is important to communicate attainable objectives. Achieving goals that may initially appear beyond a team's grasp will contribute to momentum and even greater future success, while setting goals too high might contribute to reduced morale. A good leader knows how to designate the right objective, an objective always based on discussion with team members and a desire to push toward better standards.

Rewards

Leaders are responsible for recognizing the good performance of team members. As a military leader, I often heard the Napoleonic quote, "Give me enough ribbon, and I will conquer the world," relating to the medals that he would pin on the chest of his soldiers. But in an age where every youth sport participant gets a juice box and a trophy, real leaders understand that recognition presented in the right way contributes to improved morale and a desire by participants to excel.

Not everyone should receive rewards. The best leaders set a standard to determine excellent performance before giving recognition to those who excel. A leader should never give blanket awards to everyone in the organization, as that approach devalues the actions of the most deserving. As in all leader actions, the presentation of rewards requires a keen sense of judgment and a balanced strategy.

A physician once asked me how "formal" awards should be. He then described how a team of his nurses had written him a card, telling him how much they appreciated his caring approach during a situation with a difficult patient. He wanted to reward them for their note.

A nurse overheard his question and said to him, "Doctor, don't you realize that this was their reward to *you*? They're not looking to be thanked for this; they were looking to thank you."

Formal and Informal Leaders

As basic to accomplished leaders as some of these leadership skills are, most of these techniques—setting standards, counseling, encouraging teamwork, rewarding performance, and challenging one's organization—are typically not discussed in formal medical school training.

In one PLD session, I asked a successful cardiovascular surgeon to stand. He had been performing surgery the morning of the class and had come straight from the operating room. He was still wearing scrubs. I placed an arm around his shoulder and posed a simple question to the class: "When civilians like me, without any knowledge of the intricacies of healthcare or the personalities of the various 'tribes' of physicians, walks into the hospital and sees this doctor in his scrubs with his stethoscope around his neck, what do we think? Do we see an individual dressed like this as just a doctor, or do we see something more?"

"It depends," said one seminar participant. "If he has a team around him and if he's giving instructions to some patients or a group of other hospital employees, he might be seen as a physician leader. Otherwise, he's just a doctor walking from one place in a hospital to another."

But is that true? If you had seen me in my previous job, wearing my general's stars, wouldn't you consider me a leader in the military? Almost certainly, you would. So what's the difference between an army officer with a badge of rank and a physician in scrubs? Army officers are in a profession that ascribes a leadership role to those who fit a certain description with a certain rank, no matter what job they're doing. In fact, an officer can be wearing his uniform in an airport and still be viewed by soldiers as an army leader. How does that differ from a physician wearing scrubs or a lab coat with a stethoscope? Does a doctor have to be filling a leadership slot, like a CMO or a director? Or do civilians, patients, and clinicians see physicians as leaders—*all the time?*

Doctors—because of their title, their "uniform," their knowledge, and their standing in the profession of healthcare—are by default "leaders." Whether they want to be seen that way or not makes little difference. They can be either good leaders or bad leaders, based on their attributes and competencies, but by wearing the "uniform" and having the title of "MD," they generate certain expectations. They *are* viewed as leaders.

But what about the doctor who does not serve in a formal leadership role? Who is that doctor leading?

Formal leadership is granted to individuals by virtue of job or title. The role is usually defined by a function determined by the organization, and the formal leader gets placed in a specific position of responsibility. To be placed in the position of being a formal leader requires an organization to identify specific needed competencies or requirements, and then the organization usually awards a title linked to specific expectations.

Informal leadership arises from knowledge, experience, charisma, technical expertise, or any combination of any of these that the organization considers valuable. The army has a lot of colonels, for example, but only a few of them get selected for formal leadership roles, such as commander or primary staff officer. But all of those colonels contribute in a variety of ways to build a stronger military organization.

If you're in a formal leadership position, the demands are great because you bear the responsibility for the success or failure of reaching the organization's objectives. But if you're playing an informal leadership role, you're also contributing to making the entire organization better.

Before we began the PLD seminars, I sent a letter to each individual who volunteered to be part of the inaugural course. We told participants that the key objective of the course was *not* to prepare individuals for specific leadership positions within the hospital hierarchy. They were therefore not to see the course as final preparation for individuals about to become chief medical officers or chiefs of various medical departments, institutes, or practices. Rather, we had designed the course to broaden the character and leadership abilities of all those selected to attend.

"If this course helps prepare you to lead teams and organizations and if it helps you to manage extensive responsibilities, it will be of some benefit," the letter stated. "But if it helps you to be a better physician, administrator, or clinician as you work with individual patients, their families, your healthcare teammates, or the organization, then it will be *extremely* valuable."

The same is true of this book. If what you learn in *Growing Physician Leaders* helps you to become a formal leader in some healthcare organization, great. The real goal, however, is to help you lead in healthcare, whether in some formal position or through more informal contributions.

If you're a doctor, be ready to lead!

Stages of Leading Teams

The mantle of leadership requires continuous action, assessment, understanding, involvement, communication, and energy. It also requires an understanding of how various leadership principles apply to different scenarios and specific situations.

When joining a team, leaders must first assess the existing team members and determine the current state of the team. Only after doing this and after considering a plethora of other factors can the individual best determine how to lead.

Some organizations function extremely well and need new leaders to blend into what already is taking place. Other organizations function less well and need an infusion of new blood, innovative ideas, or physicians who understand healthcare in a way that former members of the organizations did not. Leading teams already accustomed to working and communicating together in a certain way, or teams that have specific objectives already in place, requires a unique approach.

Some physician leaders will be asked to form new teams or join teams just beginning their work. On those teams, leaders have to develop new approaches to various challenges and attempt to accomplish still undetermined objectives. In these cases, physician leaders need to understand the requirements for forming teams, generating trust, and achieving results.

Forming a new team

When forming a team, a leader might have to pick key members for the team, based on an analysis of eventual objectives. After pulling the team together, the leader must immediately focus on generating trust through words, actions, and established standards. This sets the tone for all things the team eventually will be asked to do. Embodying values, keeping a professional bearing, using interpersonal tact, and creating a positive environment can quickly contribute to building trust with members of a new team.

Precise communication of standards and objectives is a critical component in establishing a solid relationship with any new team. Actively listening to new team members, showing empathy, and analyzing team members' strengths and weaknesses will greatly contribute to success. Initial counseling and continuous coaching also will give the leader a greater probability of success.

FORMING A NEW TEAM

LEADER ACTION	TEAM MEMBER REQUIREMENTS
⊙ Set the Example, Quickly Grow Trust ⊙ Communicate Objectives and Standards ⊙ Listen and Learn; Analyze Strengths and Weaknesses ⊙ Create Growth Opportunities for the Team ⊙ Refine Tasks and Responsibilities ⊙ Reward Contribution	⊙ Learn About Leader ⊙ Understand the Task, the Standards, and the Leader's Expectations ⊙ Develop Individual and Team Skills ⊙ Achieve Teamwork with Others

GENERATING TRUST IS PRIMARY REQUIREMENT

Leaders also need to understand, however, that their team members have requirements, too. In order to grow as an effective team, members must know their leader, which requires the leader to be transparent in methods, in approaches, and in his or her personality. The "led" must fully understand tasks, standards, and leader expectations. This kind of understanding requires physician leaders to provide more than an initial announcement of standards. Leaders also must take time for ongoing and continuous review of these tasks and expectations, in order to reinforce their importance.

When applied, these leadership skills allow the individual members of any new team to begin to work together. As time passes, the sense of teamwork will grow ever stronger. This occurs naturally over time with any group that comes together to accomplish some task; but to be effective and efficient, it requires the supervision of a strong leader.

Joining a "good" team already established

Forming a new team requires a unique leadership approach, as does joining a "good" team already established. The focus in this situation shifts to different attributes, competencies, and specific areas that fall under the rubric of the "seven words."

When a leader joins an established organization that has functioned for a period of time, the first leadership requirement is to determine where he or she fits. Before taking any first steps, the newly appointed leader must understand the formal and informal lines of authority, analyze the goals and objectives already set for the team, and assess how the organization runs and how the teams interact. Once the new leader makes this assessment, he or she can then proceed to build a shared trust as a member and as a leader of the team. The leader must enforce standards and make recommendations or take actions crafted to positively affect the accomplishment of objectives and bring improvement to the organization.

The first key steps to take when joining an established organization are to determine where you fit as a leader within the formal and informal hierarchy, establish how the organization is functioning, and decide how you can best contribute. At times, a leader gets placed on an established team specifically to "shake things up" or to provide a different approach to problem solving and reaching the organization's objectives. If that is the case, the nature of the assignment will influence the way the leader conducts his or her initial assessment.

JOINING A GOOD TEAM

LEADER ACTION	TEAM MEMBER REQUIREMENTS
⊙ Understand Lines of Authority	⊙ Begin to Trust New Leader
⊙ Determine Goals	⊙ Make Recommendations Affecting the Team and the New Leader
⊙ Determine Standards and Enforce Them	
⊙ Trust... and Encourage Trust	⊙ Share Information
⊙ Monitor Progress & Performance of Teams, and Adjust as Required	⊙ Cooperate with Other Team Members
⊙ Ensure Cooperation... Identify and Grow Informal Leaders and the Team	
⊙ Build Pride Through Results	

TEAM IS BUILDING COLLECTIVE PROFICIENCY

Joining a high-performing team

What typically happens when a new leader joins a high-performing team? In this situation, the new leader must first understand how his or her role will contribute to making the organization even better. Then the leader must look for ways to allow team members to achieve even greater success.

Many new leaders believe that joining and sustaining a high-performing team is the dream circumstance. But in fact, various ill-advised or hastily conceived leadership approaches—such as rashly establishing new standards, reorganizing the teams, or exerting unnecessary control—will often contribute to the team losing some of its luster. Maintaining positive momentum on a great team can be as challenging as turning around a faltering organization. It is imperative that physician leaders, many of whom will join high-performing teams, understand this.

JOINING AND SUSTAINING A GREAT TEAM

LEADER ACTION	TEAM MEMBER REQUIREMENTS
⊙ Determine Ways to Contribute	⊙ Share Mission and Values
⊙ Continue to Build Trust	⊙ Contribute to Building Greater Degrees of Trust
⊙ Focus on Polishing Team Skills and Teamwork	
	⊙ Openly Share Ideas
⊙ Quickly Respond to Issues from the Team	⊙ Assist Other Team Members in Growth
⊙ Build Pride & Spirit by Challenging (But Know Limits!)	

THE TEAM OWNS IT! THE NEW LEADER CONTRIBUTES

A Capstone Exercise

To help PLD participants build teams and accomplish organizational objectives, we wanted a capstone exercise that would challenge them to apply advanced methods of leadership. If our physician leaders were to form and lead teams, they needed to better understand the dynamics of teams, probe the motivations of others, and simultaneously apply a variety of influence techniques to multiple individuals.

We therefore conducted an in-class exercise that used a challenge the hospital actually faced, one involving the payment of physicians who respond to emergency department (ED) calls. Everyone disagreed with some element of the process or the payment model; it had been an emotional issue for the administration, emergency room physicians, and members of the hybrid medical staff "on call."

First, we described a few facts associated with "on call." We reminded our physicians of the requirements of the Federal Emergency Medical Treatment and Labor Act (EMTALA), also known as the Patient Anti-Dumping Law. EMTALA requires hospitals to provide an examination and any required stabilizing treatment, without consideration of insurance coverage or ability to pay. When a patient calls us through our Emergency Transfer Center, if we have the ability to provide care in our emergency rooms, it is the hospital's responsibility to provide it.

The population of the city of Orlando has dramatically increased in the past few years, which affects the number of patients using our emergency departments. A significant portion of ED volume is either "no pay" (those who have no medical insurance or who lack the ability to pay) or "for pay" (usually a Medicaid payment, resulting in lower billing for the same service).

AdventHealth Orlando takes patients who require specific medical attention not provided by many other hospitals in the area. While "free standing ED" services have increased throughout central Florida, those facilities often lack surgery or Intensive Care Unit capabilities. This further increases our volume and our "on call" requirements.

Every doctor with medical privileges at our hospital and who is a member of the medical staff is required to serve on call (and is paid to do so). With a significant increase in volume and an increasing "no pay" or reduced "for pay" mix, the chief financial officer has an interest in reducing this budget line, now amounting to tens of millions of dollars per year, for physicians who serve on call.

When we asked how many physicians in our PLD class were on call that day, six out of the thirty-five physicians raised their hands—but each of those physicians was affected in a different way. If a doctor is part of a practice with few partners but which receives many requests from the ED, then that physician likely will feel burdened by the call process. If a physician is part of a practice that has many partners but which does not receive many calls, then call status is more of an annoyance than a burden.

We played three actual recordings of fellow professionals answering calls from our Central Processing Center. These recorded phone conversations (part of the requirement of EMTALA) revealed physician specialists refusing to come into the hospital, not accepting patients, denying they were responsible for a transfer, or berating the young call center operator who, in every circumstance, did his federally mandated job in a professional and courteous manner. The physicians in our seminar expressed shock at the responses of their fellow professionals, but the calls presented them with a challenge: How does a leader put standards in place, and how are fellow professionals disciplined for violating those standards?

We asked four colleagues to present their point of view in regard to the state of "ED call" at AdventHealth Orlando. Then we had three actors provide the views of an established physician, a new physician to the area, and the grandmother of a patient. We asked class members, as physician leaders, to consider each of these individual's motivations.

Chief Medical Officer: *I work for two people who demand excellence in all we do. I am often called by our board of directors for an explanation of problems when we hear of patients who have not been taken care of properly or when there are serious lapses in the quality of care provided by our organization or the doctors who work with us. I'm also required to make tough calls about the medical groups we choose to associate with, how to discipline those who don't abide by our professional standards, or what direction our hospital must take in solving issues. So as you conduct an analysis of ED Call and what we have to do to make it better, please consider these things:*

First, whatever you recommend has to work... our patients must have access, we must have primary care and subspecialists respond, and we must do it in a timely manner so our patients feel they are quickly cared for and that we do it better than our competitors.

Second, we have to eliminate any issues like the ones we just heard on the call center tapes; that kind of behavior by our doctors and fellow professionals is unacceptable. We need to make sure that all the physicians on our team understand this is not our standard of care.

Finally, we have a responsibility to take care of our patients, whether they can pay us or not; an individual's insurance status will not dictate the treatment our patients receive.

Chief Clinical Officer: *It's unfortunate, but nurses get caught in the middle of doctors having these kinds of exchanges, and that's unacceptable to me. When a patient is crashing in the ED and the ED physician is saying to my nurses, "Get that specialist on the line and get him in here," my nurses don't have the time or the energy to get into a debate with a doctor. They shouldn't* *be put in the position of telling a family that a physician is on the way, when they know they are having problems getting him to the hospital. A defined call schedule is something our nurses depend on, and physicians must understand that when they are on call, they have a professional responsibility to get there when called. We have a commitment to the community to provide whatever is needed to care for patients, whether it's one a.m., six a.m., or noon.*

Chief Financial Officer: *The CEO, the COO, and the CMO all know I constantly complain about the $X million a year we spend paying doctors to do the things that I think they have a responsibility to do anyway. I hear about requests for more call pay from my financial teams and I say to myself, "How disingenuous is that? About 25 percent of the AdventHealth Orlando volume coming through the ED has no pay or Medicaid. That means 75 percent of those patients have insurance, so it seems to me you're getting paid twice in 75 percent of the cases you're supposed to be handling."*

As you can tell, this is a very frustrating topic for me, and I think there is much to be saved by the hospital in this area. Physicians won't lose anything if we do this the right way.

The ED Director (an ER physician): *I've been an ED doc in this system for fifteen years, so I've experienced some really good specialists and subspecialists who have contributed to patient care when I've called them. But truthfully, we also have some physicians who are not team players, and it's affecting our hospital's reputation and my ability to maintain effectiveness and efficiency in the ED.*

We all need to contribute to fixing this problem and making it work better, because some in our profession should be counseled

and held accountable by someone other than me. I have require-
ments from the CMO to get patient wait time down, to get a
flow through the ED, and I can't do that without your help. I
have to see all the people who come into my emergency room, but
I can't solve all their problems. I need your help with that.

The "Established Physician": *I've been around this place since*
it was a sanitarium, when it had a porch around it. But it was
much smaller when I first got here; now look at the size of this
place! If you ask me, I think there's plenty of money to go around.
I don't know why the administration is complaining about
paying for call. I've got a bunch of younger guys in my practice
who want to take call every night, and I'm more than happy to
offer them up for that service. I've got kids, and I don't have time
to do that. I don't want to do "call." I think the hospital should
pay more for us doing call, not less!

The "New Physician": *I'm a new doctor in town. I'm well trained.*
I'm enthusiastic. I'm single, so I have all the time in the world
and my nights are free. I'll just make it very easy. I will take every
call I can get, as it gives me the opportunity to improve my contact
list and my business line. And it helps me pay back my med school
loans! I will take call every night, and I will take every patient.
I don't know what the deal is with call pay, but if you pay it, I'll
take it!

The "Grandmother": *I'm going to attempt to control my*
emotions as I speak to all of you so-called doctors right now,
because I don't want to be written off as just another hysterical
grandmother. But on the inside, I'm fuming.
    When I heard from our son and daughter-in-law that there
was a medical crisis with our grandson and that they were

headed to the AdventHealth Orlando ER, I said, "You made the right decision. You will be in the very best hands. There is no better medical facility in the country. They even advertise their emergency room as being the very best on billboards all over the state. It's going to be okay."

But here it is, hours later, when I come to join them after a two-hour drive—and here they are, still sitting in the ER, with a lot of misinformation. We are not being embraced with the support we need! And we have the sense that no one is in control. We've talked to the ER doctor and many of the nurses, and they are great… but we can't seem to get a specialist on the case. Instead of feeling better about the situation, we're increasingly feeling more frightened and more anxious.

Quite frankly, our faith and trust in the organization is wavering with every minute. I would have to ask how you'd be feeling if this were your child in the ER. What would you be saying to your medical professional?

After our healthcare leaders absorbed all of this information, we gave them their task: They were to break into groups, take forty-five minutes to analyze the problem, and then reach consensus on how to build a team to successfully address the issue. They were to make sure they determined the motivations of the various individuals who had a stake in the issue and how they might influence them, based on their personalities.

We also asked them what other individuals they should consider bringing onto the team they would create. The doctors quickly concluded that they needed to bring in a lawyer, the chief of the call center, some key specialty practice leaders, and the president of the medical staff.

Finally, we asked our physician leaders to determine some short-term and long-term goals for solving the issue, along with a timeline for action.

It fascinated me to see how quickly these teams of doctors, nurses, and administrators suggested ideas to solve the problem. They honestly tried to understand the position of others, rather than just considering their own agendas, and they discussed openly how they might contribute to a proposed action plan using various forms of influence.

When we brought the teams back together, we asked none of them to describe their plans. Rather, we told them our goal had been to get them to understand how difficult it sometimes can be to build and lead teams while also gaining consensus with a group of strong-willed individuals, each holding different positions.

Leadership means having many opportunities to form and lead teams, all of them tasked with delivering solutions and making things happen. Leading teams requires passionate engagement, mutual respect, empathy, humility, team building, and purposeful communication. Great team leaders work at improving the team even as they focus on reaching organizational goals.

Whether you're a formal leader or an informal one, the same challenge applies:

Be ready to lead your team!

QUESTIONS FOR REFLECTION AND DISCUSSION

1. Identify members of your team who need either coaching or counseling. What does each of them need from you?

2. How do you use your influence methods to challenge patients, staff, and colleagues?

3. Who on your team deserves a reward? What kind of reward seems appropriate? In what context or environment should that reward be given?

4. If you are in a formal leadership role, what do you see as your primary area of responsibilities? Does your boss see it the same way? If you are in an informal leadership role, how do you support the organization and your boss?

5. Assess the team of which you're a part. Are you forming a new team, joining a good team, or sustaining a great team? How are the leaders and members of that team contributing to its success?

WAR STORY

Overcoming "Insurmountable" Challenges

So there we were...

In the winter of 1992, I found myself traveling in a small, six-passenger army jet between Washington, DC, and Fort Monroe, Virginia. I sat behind two of the army's senior leaders and got to listen in as the pair discussed the monumental organizational challenges they faced.

I took notes as my boss, General Fred Franks, the commander of the army's Training and Doctrine Command, and his boss, General Gordon Sullivan, the army's chief of staff, pondered how they would reengineer the army—an organization with 1.5 million employees and a $63 billion budget—after the fall of the Iron Curtain and the extremely successful four-day campaign called Desert Storm. They needed to transition the army from a force countering the Soviet Union in Europe to an information-age organization prepared for the demands of the twenty-first century.

At the same time, Congress was looking for a "peace dividend," concluding that the army did not need all the resources it possessed. Legislators had just told the "chief" he could reorganize however he liked, but he would need to execute a 40 percent reduction in both personnel and funding.

Though Franks and Sullivan had very different personalities, both were dedicated professionals, intellectually gifted, terrific leaders, and selfless patriots. They had fought together in Vietnam, served as comrades on multiple occasions in Europe during the Cold War, and had fought as a team during Desert Storm. While Franks fought on the battlefields of Iraq and Kuwait, Sullivan fought on the military-political front in DC, supporting his friend in the conflict. As engaged historians, they both knew how leaders of America's army had failed in the past when facing these kinds of challenges. They refused to permit failure again.

"Dammit, Freddie, some are clamoring for us to just bring the force down—cut troops and money, without thinking of the threats our country faces now or will face in the future. We can't let that happen," Sullivan declared. "We've got to organize and understand how to do this smartly. If anyone thinks we're just going to be caretakers of a smaller army, we're going to have to prove them wrong. We need to reduce unnecessary overhead, and we need to change the way we do things. We need to make our army smaller, but it still has to be ready to fight."

While doing all of this, the two men knew they could not lose the trust of their fellow soldiers. They also knew the paramount importance of their mission: defend the country and provide security for their fellow citizens. At the same time, they also needed to continuously modernize equipment to keep overmatching capabilities against potential threats; provide funds for critical personnel, maintenance, and training requirements; and find new ways to counter emerging threats, all while continuing to support new ways to deploy and station soldiers in places where they needed to remain. A tall order!

After listening to these old friends on that short plane ride discuss the challenges they faced, it struck me that they and the army were facing impossible odds and insurmountable obstacles. But then I watched as together they began energetically hatching a multifaceted plan, listing every possible problem and how they might solve each one. They decided to form "teams of teams" as part of an overarching campaign plan, enlisting experts with complementary personalities, placing them under the right subordinate leaders, succinctly defining their tasks and then providing them with a vision for the objectives they had to achieve. They held all their teams in suspense, making the leaders responsible while closely monitoring their progress and keeping a hand on the rheostat of challenge.

While managing the various aspects of the plan might seem overwhelming, the two generals knew their top priority was leading the force: building trust, keeping organizational values strong, constantly engaging all the elements of the team. They would expand their travel schedule and visit forces all over the world; personally communicate their vision using every means available; and find new ways to engage, empower, and energize subordinate leaders to ensure a common understanding of objectives at every level, while also encouraging constructive dissent and investing in the development of people and organizations. Their brilliant plan combined their inherent soldier skills, learned management techniques, and energetic leadership methods.

I learned that day that overcoming the seemingly insurmountable challenges of organizations, especially large ones, requires skill, adept management of others, and creative leadership.

CHAPTER 7

Those Idiots at Higher Headquarters

I n the army, when a breakdown in communication or a deficiency in understanding occurs between the "executives" and the soldiers they lead, we use a tongue-in-cheek expression to describe the disconnect: "Those idiots at higher headquarters just don't get it!" Any soldier in a foxhole, fighting off the enemy in lousy weather with the odds apparently stacked against him, will find it easy to use this derisive statement to explain the obvious stupidity of those in the rear area, viewing their maps and plans in a well-lit, environmentally safe zone. Those "idiots at higher headquarters" plainly have no clue about what's really going on!

But when soldiers (or subordinate leaders) continue to grow in their leadership journey, they acquire greater insight into the intricacies of the plan and how they fit in. They gain a greater understanding of, and sometimes even an appreciation for, the decisions made by those in the rear. In doing so, they realize that, just maybe, those guys at higher headquarters really aren't so dumb after all.

157

Part of Something Bigger

Leading as part of a larger organization can look quite different than leading from a foxhole (or from an office in the hospital, some distance from the chief executive officer). Regardless of position, rank, or status, emerging leaders eventually will have an epiphany related to their role as a part of something "bigger."

Early in a career, emerging leaders tend to keep a singular focus on their group of subordinates. They concentrate strongly on accomplishing the mission immediately in front of them, and so they soon learn that the motivations of their followers and the influence techniques they use will help them to reach their goals. As they grow, however, they gradually take on a more strategic view of the whole organization. In doing so, they come to recognize, and then to understand, their particular leadership role within a much larger organization.

No matter their position, someone will always outrank them. Someone will always have a better view of the direction of the organization and how groups within that organization can best help the whole achieve its goals.

In the military, an individual might rise to the exalted position of chairman of the Joint Chiefs. The selectee for this position holds four-star rank, represents all uniformed services, and serves as the nation's top military official. The chairman leads the Joint Staff; builds consensus among the service chiefs of the army, navy, air force, and marines; and coordinates the actions of uniformed commanders all over the globe. He also contributes as part of the president's national security team.

Most importantly, the chairman knows he is part of a bigger team, which requires that he understand the national security structure—the State Department, the Congress, Homeland Security, Treasury, CIA, etc.—as well as the inner workings of the military.

In a similar way, young physician leaders in charge of specific teams must remember that they may also rise to higher, more formal positions in their practice, at their hospital, in a healthcare network, or in healthcare writ large. For that reason, they must grasp how to be part of a bigger organization while still leading at their current level.

To lead healthcare organizations, physicians must understand how to influence, and equally as important, how they will be influenced by, the goals of the organizations to which they belong. To accomplish this, physicians must gain insight into the goals, executive decision-making processes, and some of the strategy that drives the approach of their particular healthcare organization.

While plenty of schools teach marketing, strategy, finance, and business design, such formal courses often don't address the pragmatics of particular markets or specialized healthcare visions. Growing physician leaders need to see more of what goes on behind the curtain at their organizations to better understand the desired connection between the science of healing and the art of healthcare.

If our experience at AdventHealth is any indication, many physicians do not know the strategy, direction, or objectives of their hospitals or institutions. The relationship between the institution's administration and the medical staff, representing several groups, specialties, and practices, often gets hampered by miscommunication from both sides. Physicians often claim passionately that the organization's executives "just don't get it" on key healthcare issues. At AdventHealth, many physicians wondered if the true objective of the PLD course was to convince the doctors to "get in line with the hospital's directives." That kind of thinking indicates the level of distrust that often exists at many institutions, from physicians to administrators and from executives back to physicians.

Much of this frustration has its roots in misunderstanding and insufficient communication, due largely to a lack of knowledge about the strategic direction of a hospital and the workings of its executive administration. That's an unfortunate phenomenon, not at all unique to AdventHealth or to any large organization. And the best way to address the problem is to explore what the organization does for doctors, and then investigate what doctors can do for the organization. Let's look at each in turn.

What Any Organization Does for Doctors

Not surprisingly, many doctors, because they're busy taking care of patients, remain unaware of the strategy, vision, and direction of their organization. At the same time, many executives do not take the time to include physicians in discussions regarding the strategic approach of the organization. But to be an integral part of the team that drives change, physicians must understand what the "idiots at higher headquarters" are doing, and executives need to do a better job of including physicians in key discussions.

To help our own PLD participants understand their place in the larger organization, we invited three top administrators to speak to the group about their role in helping the institution to succeed. Their presentations allowed our front line physician leaders to better understand, many for the first time, how they might, as part of the team and as leaders within the team, contribute to the accomplishment of the hospital's goals and objectives. While the administrators' comments pertain specifically to AdventHealth and its operations, the vast majority of their remarks apply equally to healthcare at large.

The Chief Operating Officer

Brian Paradis serves as the chief operating officer of AdventHealth Orlando. Armed with an accounting degree and a mastery of financial details, he formerly served as the hospital's chief financial officer as it grew into the healthcare behemoth it now is in Central Florida. Brian cares passionately for the twenty-two thousand employees of the organization and has a keen understanding of how people, systems, and processes contribute to the effectiveness and efficiency of the hospital. A self-proclaimed introvert and deep thinker, he also is a compelling and engaging leader as he focuses continually on ways to build consensus. Hospital staff and physicians alike admire his leadership and his vision for the organization.

Brian once was asked to speak at a national healthcare conference. He followed a CEO from another hospital who obviously felt proud of his organization. The man introduced himself by spending an excessive amount of time touting the capabilities and buildings of his facility: its number of beds, its multi-specialty services, and the credentials of its newly hired doctors. As Brian listened, he realized he needed to adjust his own presentation. To open his talk in front of hundreds of healthcare executives, he said simply, "I'm Brian Paradis. I'm from AdventHealth Orlando, and we love taking care of people."

In the early stages of his career as an accountant, Brian focused on the financial bottom line. But soon it became apparent to him that most great businesses succeed by improving their product. Given that a hospital's "product" is the patient, it made sense to Brian that the core processes associated with patient care, not marketing or financials, should be the driving force in building a successful organization.

"It was funny," Brian said. "I took over as the COO and I went to conferences where I heard a lot of people in healthcare talking about market share and financial concerns. I could not, for the life of me, understand why organizations delivering healthcare don't talk all that much about their patients, or why executives don't have a common language and a common frame of reference with those who work on the 'product.' Other than the CMO and the chief clinical officer, I saw very few people walking around the clinical space who were asking folks, 'Do you have what you need? Do you know how we're performing? Do we know what you still need from us?' Until everyone starts to think that way, then we're missing the chance to be a great team. Executives and administrators need to find ways to more effectively team with healthcare providers, and healthcare providers need to find ways to more effectively team with us. We need to understand each other's languages."

Because the "experts" in treating patients are physicians and clinicians, and not marketers and administrators, Brian believes that pulling physicians into the institution's leadership team will help the hospital perform better, resulting in better patient care. He also believes that everything "interesting" in patient care relates to team interaction and that all pieces of the team should come together under great leaders to ensure the product (the patient) receives the best care possible.

For Brian, big ideas start with convictions. The first conviction of our organization is linked to the AdventHealth mission: "Extend the healing ministry of Christ." This requires excellence from everyone as measured by common medical standards, and then to do even more because the mission demands it.

Brian believes that although most doctors will spend little of their time working with the mental and social side of their patients, and even less on the spiritual side, when they understand that human beings consist of three primary components—physical, mental/social, and spiritual—then they can begin to see why AdventHealth must extend its care to the whole person. "We want to go beyond healing sick people," he said. "We want to help restore people to their fullest potential. That should be what makes us different—and it will take a true team to do that."

Many professionals in our class had never heard how the strategy, the vision, and the mission of AdventHealth all tie together with specific action. After hearing Brian's talk, they began to make the connection between the growth and strength of our organization and how they, as physicians, could best serve their patients.

While many COOs likely provide similar addresses on the growth and health of their organizations to a variety of audiences, including their boards of directors, Brian chose to address his physician leaders. "We need a stronger, more fully spread core of physicians who understand what we can do together," he declared. "Then that core of physicians will need to lead their colleagues and peers in how we best care for people. We have made an investment in training physicians to be healthcare leaders, and we want them to help us lead this organization. We're headed down the rapids toward some really interesting water. We can figure out how to steer the boat, but we need leaders among our physicians to tell us where the big boulders are. Together we'll navigate this, but we can't do it without our physicians as an integral part of the team."

Marketing and Business Strategies

As senior vice president for strategic planning at AdventHealth, Dr. Josef Ghosn serves as our primary marketing strategist. Conscientious and with a penchant for detail, Josef is exceedingly smart, engaging, and personable. The little that remains of his Lebanese accent contributes to a dry and disarming sense of humor. His ability to weave amusing stories into discussions of the practical application of business theory make him an engaging speaker.

Josef gave our physicians insight into healthcare's new growth paradigm with a view toward what future growth might look like in our market area. He spoke of healthcare "supply and demand" and the various ways of reacting to those trends: pricing and volume models related to Medicare, Medicaid, insurance, no-pay, and the effects of the Affordable Care Act (ACA); the uniqueness of the various markets which our eight hospitals serve and the demographics associated with each; and an analysis of how emergency department visits translate into requirements for physician specialty services.

It amazes many physicians to see a pragmatic business analysis of the areas of their practice. They often don't realize how the hospital uses that information to help physicians provide the best focused care for patients, while simultaneously helping doctors to succeed in their practices.

Josef emphasized that continued growth and success must be earned. Changes relating to the ACA, price and payment, supply and demand, and healthcare insurance issues mean doctors and hospitals will have to adapt the old model they once relied upon. In the future, the success and growth of hospitals and individual physician practices will depend on choice—getting chosen by patients, payers, managed care companies, employers, and a variety of others—by virtue of the quality, price, services, the patient experience, teamwork, and leadership they offer.

Josef provided emerging market information that ran the gamut from the role and success of urgent care facilities and freestanding emergency departments to cooperation with large industry worksite wellness sites and clinics that address prevention, pre-acute and post-acute care, as well as acute care. He gave an update on the various brick-and-mortar specialty institutes we had created, the research program we had established, the translational tools we had incorporated, and the training and leader development model we believe will contribute to better effectiveness and efficiency. He revealed the world of the hospital to them in business terms, a world most doctors never get to see.

Hospital executives had agreed, Josef said, that government policy change related to the ACA would be profound but gradual. He affirmed the hospital administration's belief that there will always be choice in America and that the kind of universal healthcare that exists in countries such as Sweden, Norway, France, and others will not be implemented in our country. Exchanges will continue, but always with an element of choice.

In the future, healthcare will have to find ways to treat all patients with a form of standardized and masterful care, delivered with excellence as perceived by patients. Hospitals like ours, because of their tax-exempt, faith-based approach and unique mission, will have to bring improved treatment to the underserved.

As hospitals plan for the future, they will need to address all factors along a continuum of care: prevention, pre-acute, acute, post-acute, and aged care. Hospitals can no longer focus only on "healing." They must instead build a lasting relationship over a lifetime with patients and their families.

Josef also predicted that fee-for-service will see significant reductions as a primary method of charging patients. Payment mechanisms are already in place for quality and performance, and over the next few years, they will continue to grow in scope and complexity, including both government and private payers. The detailed elements of a pay-for-performance approach will naturally evolve as organizations continue to grapple with growing healthcare costs and improved processes for the delivery of services.

While Josef's comments were quite specific to what was happening at the time, the main point I wanted to make with our physicians as they listened to Josef is that hospital administrators often conduct extensive analysis on market conditions in an effort to help the organization make better decisions. Too often, physicians don't understand or see how such market analysis behind the scenes are contributing to their success "in the trenches" of healthcare.

In the past, hospital goals and physician goals were seldom coordinated or aligned. Josef insisted that this must change. Physician-hospital alignment is critical to the success of both groups, as well as to the future of effective healthcare in this country. The two parties must work together to apply standards in all practices and processes. All our physicians agreed.

Chief Clinical Officer

Sheryl Dodds, AdventHealth Orlando's chief clinical officer, is one of the more charismatic leaders in our organization. In her quest to identify ways to improve healthcare, she continuously wanders around the organization, searching for new ideas and ways to improve the team. She's an excellent coach and trainer, and her pleasant demeanor sometimes hides her focus on holding her nurses to exacting standards. Sheryl informed our physician leaders about several clinical initiatives but focused on two that she leads: CREATION Life and patient experience.

CREATION Life is a wellness philosophy based on a holistic health approach. The acronym CREATION stands for Choice, Rest, Environment, Activity, Trust, Interpersonal Relationships, Outlook, and Nutrition. While most organizational health and wellness programs focus primarily on exercise and diet, the CREATION Life approach takes into account multiple factors that contribute to better emotional, spiritual, and physiological well-being. The CREATION Life philosophy was applied to the architectural design and construction of one of our newer hospitals, built on Disney property across from the Magic Kingdom and Disney's Experimental Prototype Community of Tomorrow (EPCOT). Disney's executives sponsored a competition for healthcare organizations to design a hospital for its experimental town of Celebration; it also asked contestants to pattern their facility on how healthcare should look in the future. They asked the question, "How would you create the healthiest community in America?" The AdventHealth vision won, AdventHealth Celebration went up on the south side of Orlando, and the holistic health concept of CREATION Life became the foundation for the flagship facility.

Sheryl came to AdventHealth Orlando shortly after the Disney event took place, joining us after running a cardiac care hospital in Nebraska. When she saw a book about CREATION Life and noticed banners, placards, and other marketing tools about it all around the hospital, she asked, "How is this affecting our patients? What are we doing with this philosophy? What is the true meaning of each of those letters, and how can we incorporate it into patient care?"

She thought the hospital could do more with this approach, even making it the organization's central approach to care. "If we're taking care of the whole patient," she said, "if, as a nurse or a caregiver, you really want to help that person regain their full potential, then we need to do more than just take care of our patients' physical needs and heal them. They need to understand their choices for personal growth. They need to understand the importance of rest, not just for the body, but also for the soul. They need to learn how to create a healthy environment in their home and work space that will help them to thrive. They need to understand the connection between spirituality and health. They need to grasp how their mental attitude and outlook affects their well-being. And they need to understand that strong relationships contribute to a healthy body, mind, and spirit."

Under Sheryl's leadership, the clinical teams, primarily the nurse care managers, developed tools and various processes to help integrate the CREATION Life principles across our facilities to provide a guide for addressing patients and to give those patients a better understanding of their treatment methodologies. The process now has been standardized across all our hospitals and campuses.

After leading this charge, Sheryl then recognized she'd made a mistake. Like many executives and administrators, she realized she had left doctors out of the loop. She took advantage of the Physician Leader Development course to engage leaders who could introduce the concept to the body of physicians comprising our AdventHealth family.

Sheryl also told our doctors that healthcare providers across America are notorious for being part of a population that does not take care of itself, whether physically, emotionally, or spiritually. Many doctors and nurses suffer from the same maladies as the patients they treat, although most of them do not get the same kind of help. Across the board, healthcare providers are sleep deprived; and because of shift requirements and call, they do not eat or exercise well. As they nurture others and dispense advice on any number of wellness issues, many healthcare providers do not set the kind of example that can inspire their patients. "Especially nurses," Sheryl said, being kind to the doctors in the room who also suffered the same malaise.

Part of the CREATION Life approach requires the employees of AdventHealth—doctors, nurses, technicians, and administrators—to become models of holistic health. CREATION Life recently began a focused employee health and wellness model that is gaining popularity across the hospital campuses.

Sheryl also informed our physicians about hospital issues relating to patient experience. She described the way the administration and the clinical staff had analyzed HCAHPS (Hospital Consumer Assessment of Healthcare Provider and Systems) areas, and how they were attempting to improve in each of those areas. Again, she admitted they had not included physicians as part of the team when her clinicians developed methods to better meet the expectations of patients (and as a result, the Physician Communication component of the HCAHPS of Patient Experience continues to lag behind other areas, which are showing improvement).

"I've been a nurse for many years," Sheryl said, "and sometimes it's hard for us to ask doctors to help with projects that all of us know will improve healthcare, because we know how busy you are with your patients. But I've learned something in watching this group over the last few months. You are busy, but you want to be involved. We should not hesitate to ask you to be a part of the team, and you should not hesitate to lead the teams, because you all have so much to contribute!"

Maybe They Aren't Such Idiots?

At the end of this session, the PLD participants had a better situational awareness of what the executives, administrative team, and support staff of AdventHealth do in terms of developing strategy, creating vision, and maintaining organizational structure. One of the physicians who coincidentally, like me, is a huge baseball fan, spoke up and made this analogy:

You know, I'm starting to see a hospital is a lot like a profess-ional baseball team. When you're at a game, it's easy to focus on just the "stars" of the team—the players out on the field. You might have a pitcher throwing incredible hundred-mile-an-hour fastballs or a batter knocking home runs out of the park that garners your attention. That's what makes baseball exciting. But there are plenty of other people doing a whole lot of work in the background so the stars of the team can shine.

Think about it. Every successful ball club has a general manager developing a farm team. The owner builds a stadium and generates an excitement about the hometown team. The groundskeepers prepare the field. The director of admissions manages ticket sales. The concessions crew orders enough food and drinks for the fans. There are thousands who con-tribute to the success of the team, but they're not the ones who get all the attention. Yet without them, that superstar pitcher or home run hitter is just standing out there playing a game.

Those star pitchers and batters in baseball are a lot like doctors in healthcare. Doctors perform critical work, they're often at the center of attention, and frequently thought of as the "stars" of medicine. But they can't do their work alone. They need visionaries building hospitals. Administrators running them. Billing directors handling finances. Environmental services keeping spaces clean. Nurses caring for patients. Plus someone contributing to the thousand other things that go into making a hospital successful. Without everybody contributing in their own special area, the healing doesn't take place as effectively or as successfully.

Heads nodded as the doctor finished. In the discussion that followed, one concept became clear. Participants in our PLD course were beginning to see they needed insight into the goals, executive decision-making processes, and some of the strategy that drive the running of their hospital. They now had a better understanding, many for the first time, of how they were part of the team. And with that greater understanding, they realized that maybe, just maybe, those idiots at higher headquarters weren't so dumb after all.

QUESTIONS FOR REFLECTION
AND DISCUSSION

1. What are the goals, objectives, and strategies of your organization? How do you contribute to these?

2. What strategic initiatives exist in your healthcare institution? Are physician insights contributing to advances or problem solving? If not, how can you "lead up" to be included in the discussion?

3. What is your organization doing to promote exceptional holistic health as the basis for all other forms of excellence and to prevent physician burnout? Since you are committed to excellence, what plan do you have to increase your own health and fitness?

WAR STORY

Take Us Down the Right Path

So there we were...

In the spring of 1986, I was in the final year of a three-year tour as an instructor at the US Military Academy. Like many other captains, the army had sent me for a master's degree in exercise physiology to prepare for a three-year teaching assignment in the Department of Physical Education at West Point. The army calls this kind of posting a professional "broadening assignment," but the assignment at this beautiful location in upstate New York also provided some much-needed family time after ten years in the operational army.

As the cadets prepared for their spring break that year, my wife thought we should plan a short family excursion with our two small boys. Sue always looked for ways to combine outdoor fun with some sort of educational experience for our sons, so our vacations usually took on a combination of travel, activity, and learning. I had recently finished Michael Shaara's *The Killer Angels*, an excellent historical novel on the Civil War. I had recounted several of my favorite passages to her and the boys over dinner. One night, she asked if I had ever been to Gettysburg, the setting of the battle described in the book. I told her that I hadn't, but she surprised me when she reported she had, as a young child, with her parents and grandparents.

"Mark," she said one evening, "you need to go there. It was such a long time ago, but I remember it as such a beautiful and pastoral place. Even though I was only about six years old, I remember this giant map in a big auditorium, with different colored lights that showed the movement of forces and how the battle evolved. It's a great part of our history, and as a military guy, you really ought to see it. Plus, the boys would enjoy all the cannons around the fields and they'd be able to work off some energy, running around."

Sue wanted to visit a battlefield? I felt skeptical. In addition, the campaigns of the Civil War never interested me much, despite my military career. I had earned mediocre grades in the mandatory "History of the Military Art" courses I'd taken as a cadet a decade earlier, and of all the history we studied, the campaigns of the Civil War seemed the most confusing to me. Like most Americans, I could name Grant, Lee, and Jackson as key leaders, but in my view, a trip to a Civil War battlefield as a family vacation didn't sound terribly exciting. While I admitted *The Killer Angels* was a great read, I recognized it as more a flowing piece of fiction than a boring military account.

But since Sue had already energized our two young sons, it looked like we would be heading to Gettysburg. We planned a few days of leave (vacation), reserved a cheap hotel room, gassed up the minivan, loaded our excited five- and seven-year-old boys, and headed for Adam's County, Pennsylvania.

Sue went into high gear to prepare for the trip. In every educational experience for our boys, she found ways to make learning fun. While I had a brief recollection of the Gettysburg campaign from my time as a cadet, she started researching the battle and began piecing together fun facts to impress Todd and Scott. The several-hour drive passed quickly as she recounted to the boys some of her "fun history."

She would show them a map and then cite some bizarre fact she had discovered about the battle. "Did you know," she began, "that West Point—where we live—was very important in producing leaders for the Civil War? There were sixty major battles, and in fifty-five of them, West Point graduates commanded the army on both sides! And in the other five, West Pointers commanded on at least one side. At Gettysburg, eighty-three West Point generals were on the field, nearly evenly distributed on both sides. Some of these men fought against their best friends!"

I had heard this kind of propaganda from my colleagues in the History Department (they liked quoting their unofficial motto: "Much of the history we teach was made by the people we taught!"), but the kids seemed both enthralled and mesmerized. It amazed me that my bride had found so many interesting facts.

After checking in to our hotel, we quickly walked the few blocks to the park's visitor center. The giant map with all the lights that once had made such an impression on my wife was still there. We settled into our seats in a bowl-shaped auditorium to hear the thirty-minute presentation. The lights dimmed and the utterly fascinating presentation enthralled boys and father alike. The lights and commentary managed to hold the rapt attention of our two normally fidgeting youngsters. And the moving parts, the flow of forces, the approach by leaders, the elements of strategy and tactics I had never before considered also kept my attention.

The geographic nature of the battlefield surprised me. Not counting the approaching roads (or the scene of the cavalry fight on the third day, which occurred several miles east of town), the battle raged on undulating terrain crisscrossed by roads and Pennsylvania farm fences in an area about eight kilometers long from north to south and five kilometers wide from east to west. The battle tore across fields sown with crops, fruit orchards, partitioned farmland, steep hills, dense wood, rocky outcropping, creeks, and marshes. The small city of Gettysburg sat at the convergence of eight roads, smack dab in the middle of the fight. The battle unfolded over three days in this highly contained area, with more than one hundred thousand soldiers in blue and gray taking part. It became one of the bloodiest battles of the war.

As we left the map presentation, Sue and I discussed how to best drive around the battlefield. A young national park ranger heard us talking and asked what type of car we drove. A minivan, we replied. "Well," she said, "if you don't mind paying a small fee, we have certified battlefield tour guides who can drive the tricky roads around here and give you a tour at the same time." Even on a captain's pay, that sounded like a great deal.

A few minutes later, an older park ranger approached our car. Avuncular and wearing a huge smile, he introduced himself: "Ranger Tim... all of you, call me Ranger Tim! I'm proud of being a national park ranger, and I'm honored to help you learn more about your American history at what I believe is the most beautiful and sacred place on all the earth." He asked whether we had ever visited Gettysburg and then sought permission to drive our car during the tour.

For the next three hours, we wove through the streets, the roads, and the dirt trails of Gettysburg National Park. Ranger Tim pointed out statues and described in loving detail what they represented. He shared stories of the men who had fought at the various places we stopped, using their own words. He continuously read copies of letters they had written home to loved ones that he pulled from the oversized knapsack he kept on the floor between driver and passenger. He spoke the words of generals, privates, and sergeants. Ranger Tim's voice became soft when he told emotional stories about the people involved, and yet his voice also boomed when he imitated the sounds of battlefield chaos, like the roar of the cannons, the whinnying of the horses, the crack of a sniper's round. We laughed at some of his antics and sound effects, and I became emotional on several occasions as I thought about those who gave their lives on this sacred ground.

Ranger Tim took us to McPherson Ridge, where the battle began on July 1, 1863. We then spent time on the top of wooded Culp's Hill, where the battle raged for three uninterrupted days. Ranger Tim spent a significant amount of time explaining General Longstreet's countermarch along Seminary Ridge on the second day of the battle, as this southern genius approached and attempted to outflank the increasingly robust Union force under General Meade, piecemealed onto Cemetery Ridge. Ranger Tim allowed the boys to play on the boulders thrown about Devil's Den, run through the fruit trees of the Peach Orchard, and climb the rocky hill at the front of Little Round Top. But each time he started to tell another story, they sat enthralled by the words and the mannerisms of this man who obviously loved what he was doing as a history teacher and as a keeper of a nation's saga.

We were scheduled to finish at The Angle, that piece of ground called the high water mark of the Confederacy. At this place, the clash of northern and southern troops grew so intense on July 3 that the state of the Union hung in the balance for a few seconds. In the end, the north prevailed. All Americans should have the experience of standing on that ground.

"Well, it's been wonderful this afternoon with you," Ranger Tim said, another huge smile directed to our two adoring boys. Then he turned to us. "Mom and Dad, would you like one more extra stop, one that I only give to special people?"

"Of course!" we both said excitedly.

"Well, okay then," Ranger Tim replied, "but you have to be real quiet and not say a word."

We walked across the visitor center parking lot and through the gates of the Gettysburg National Cemetery on the hill overlooking the town. We silently walked down the gravel path until our guide suddenly stopped and pointed to a spot on the ground. He startled us by turning around quickly, as if he had discovered something he had searched for over many years.

"It was right here, we think," he said quietly. "The grandstand was right here, where President Lincoln came almost four months after the last bullet was fired. Even though it was November, they were still burying the bodies that had been lying in the fields from the fight the previous summer. Mr. Lincoln wasn't the key speaker on November 19. That honor was bestowed on Edward Everett, who spoke for almost two hours. No one really remembered what he said. But Mr. Lincoln's remarks lasted about two minutes, and everyone to this day remembered what he said."

Then Ranger Tim began reciting the Gettysburg Address, right there, as if he were channeling our great president. Other tourists who had been walking through the grounds started gathering around us, listening as intently as we were to this park ranger. He spoke as if he were in a trance. When he finished, he looked directly into the eyes of our two boys.

"I hope you learned some things today, and I hope no matter what you do in the future, you'll be a leader for our country and take us down the right path. That's what Mr. Lincoln would've wanted."

He tousled their hair and then headed back to the visitor's center without saying goodbye or looking back.

CHAPTER 8

Becoming Physicians Who Transform Healthcare

L eadership makes a difference. A *huge* difference.

Good leadership paves the way for success and good outcomes, while poor leadership can condemn good people to failure and tragic outcomes. We see this scenario replayed every day in every arena of life.

Since I spent so many years of my life in the military, however, and since good and poor leadership tends to produce such stark results on the battlefield, to this day when I want to bring to life lessons on leadership such as those we've surveyed in this book, I like to take people to the wonderful national park known as Gettysburg.

Doctors on a Battlefield

Thousands of books have been written about the Battle of Gettysburg. Several movies also have depicted the critical action that took place

179

from July 1–3, 1863. The most popular film, *Gettysburg*, produced in 1993 by Ted Turner, was based on the highly acclaimed and easy-to-read historical novel I read before visiting Gettysburg, *The Killer Angels* by Michael Shaara. Both the film and the novel focus on a few interesting characters and their decisive actions during the fight.

To put a capstone on our Physician Leader Development course, we invited all fifty participants to come with us to Gettysburg and to experience what in the military we call a "battle staff ride." We required those who made the trip (forty-seven out of fifty) to read *The Killer Angels*, and most of our physician leaders also watched *Gettysburg*.

But we asked them to do more.

More than one hundred thousand men took the field of battle during the critical three days of early July 1863. Several thousand formal leaders, and many more informal ones, contributed to the action and to the outcome. With all these personalities, history gives us scores of leadership stories to tell, so we employed the staff ride technique of role-playing.

We wanted to use this amazing outdoor classroom to drive home the critical elements of leadership that our physicians had discovered over the previous several months. We would analyze human interaction under stressful conditions, discuss concepts linked to team building and formation of organizational behaviors, and would find additional ways to help doctors learn from soldiers. Then we would apply those battlefield lessons to healthcare issues.

The bonus was that we would have a lot of fun doing it.

Origin of the Battle Staff Ride

You've probably never heard of Eben Swift, but I love the guy. The son of an army surgeon, he was born in 1854 in Texas but studied at Racine College in Wisconsin, at Washington University in St. Louis, and at

Dickinson College in Carlisle, Pennsylvania, before receiving a degree and a commission in 1876 from the United States Military Academy.

As a new lieutenant, his service began on the Indian frontiers of Wyoming, Montana, Nebraska, Idaho, and Colorado against the Sioux, Cheyenne, Barrock, and Ute Indians. Later, during the Spanish-American War, he helped prepare parts of Puerto Rico for civil government. He saw combat against the Moros in the Philippines, served as an observer in Manchuria during the Russo-Chinese War, and commanded a cavalry regiment in the 1916 punitive expedition in Mexico. He helped organize the famous "Rainbow Division" before it headed to France for World War I and then commanded US forces in Italy before he retired as a major general in May 1918.

After retirement, the army called him back to become an instructor of tactics and military history at the War College. Teaching was his passion.

To be sure, Swift distinguished himself as an eclectic soldier. But an innovation he developed as a young major in 1906, while teaching at the Command and Staff College at Leavenworth, Kansas, really captures my attention.

Swift thought it important for his students to see military history as more than just the outcome of battles and campaigns. In what we might call an "adult learning model," Swift wanted his students to study, and then experience, the complex association between the personalities and emotions of the leaders, the effects of the environment, and a sound application of theory. So he designed what he would call a "battle staff ride."

In the summer of 1906, he and twelve student officers boarded a train in Kansas bound for Georgia, for the sole purpose of walking the grounds of a Civil War battlefield. For years afterward, the staff ride was viewed as the most exciting part of the curriculum. But then Major Swift left for a new assignment and other subjects began to intrude on the program.

"Staff riding" got rejuvenated in the '60s and '70s, and then formalized once more in 1982–83, as part of a curriculum at Ft. Leavenworth...

only a few years before newly promoted Major Mark Hertling would take the course.

With fond memories of our family's emotional experience with the park ranger at Gettysburg, I signed up for the elective. I found it a fascinating way to study the complexities of leadership and decision making, as well as a unique way to build teams. That was the first of many staff rides I would take in years to come.

After graduating from Leavenworth and getting assigned to Europe as the First Armored Division Chief of Operations, one of my first tasks was to develop a staff ride for the senior leaders of the division. With the help of Professor and head of the West Point History Department, Colonel (now retired Brigadier General) Robert Doughty, we took leaders to the Ardennes battlefields near Sedan, Belgium, and used that theater to discuss the initial phases of World War I. That was the first of more than forty battlefield staff rides I experienced with operational units that I either led or was a part of, and these rides became key ingredients for the leader development programs of many organizations.[15]

Despite their beautiful scenery, however, the battlefields of Europe are not well marked. In fact, many of the buildings and roads have changed so markedly that individuals seeking lessons from their history must assess old maps, analyze unit historical records, and guess at the location of the battles that took place there. That may be because Europe has suffered so many wars on the same ground; countless leadership lessons have been learned and relearned over the millennia.

But Gettysburg is different. The staff rides there are my favorite. The National Park Service does a magnificent job of maintaining the parks, and in the early part of the twentieth century, so many veteran organizations wanted to honor their units and their heroes that the battlefield has become a treasure trove of monuments of all sizes, shapes, and designs. An amateur historian, or someone interested in the Civil War, can spend a whole day traveling the forests, dens, hills, pastures, and rock formations of this small town in Adams County and walk away with a better understanding of what happened there. In my view, every American should have this experience, because the sacred ground of Gettysburg has such a critical place in our history. And if you want to learn more about leadership… that is there, too.

It isn't just military history that visitors can find at Gettysburg. The battleground also provides valuable insight into countless issues linked to human interaction, leader engagement, organizational strengths, and dysfunction and task completion. The Army War College's Carlisle Foundation believes it offers so much more than military lessons that it established a program in the 1990s for Fortune 500 companies to bring their executives to learn history, strategy, and leadership by touring Gettysburg under the tutelage of War College professors. While every visitor to Gettysburg walks away with a better understanding of an important piece of American history, a battle ride also serves as a powerful classroom for anyone wanting to improve their leadership skills and understanding of organizational strategy.

Preparing for Gettysburg

We scheduled our Gettysburg ride for August and assigned characters in April, to allow plenty of time for research. We asked each participant to research their assigned individual's personality and contribution to the fight.

Our class didn't know this in advance, but during the ride, we would call on participants to provide information about their character. They would then interact with other characters regarding their view of what was happening, as compared to what others saw and the actions others took. The interactive nature of the staff ride places each role player in the position of understanding his or her character, while also forcing unrehearsed interaction with others. While we didn't want to turn our physician leaders into either amateur historians or part-time soldiers, we did want them to learn about the attributes and the characteristics of leadership represented by each character.

To make this event really come alive, we worked with our professional historian, Colonel Doug Douds, a marine on a teaching assignment at the Army's War College at Carlisle, to assign character roles to our students. We wanted to "channel" specific personalities at several different "stands"—staff ride talk for locations on the ground where some specific action took place—to generate discussion about the effects of leadership.

Colonel Douds brought a dry sense of humor and a fun-loving charisma to his vast knowledge of history and of the Gettysburg battle personalities. A marine F/A-18 fighter pilot, Doug had flown combat sorties off aircraft carriers over Bosnia, Kosovo, and Iraq and had served peacetime deployments in Japan, Korea, Thailand, and the Philippines. As a graduate of the navy's Fighter Weapons School (Top Gun), he also had attended the army's War College at Carlisle, Pennsylvania, right up the road from Gettysburg. Doug is a soldier-scholar; while an expert in war fighting skills, he also served as part of the Commander's Action Group, a type of internal think tank in the Pentagon, for two chairmen of the Joint Chiefs. Following his Pentagon assignment, and facing what he knew would be retirement from his beloved Marine Corps, he returned to Carlisle for one final tour to teach the Advanced Strategic Art Program at the Army War College.

A Pennsylvanian by birth and the son of a Division II college football coach (who recently passed Lou Holtz on the all-time games won list), Doug first visited the Gettysburg battlefield when he was ten years old. He got hooked. While other kids collected baseball cards or seashells, Doug collected books and anecdotes of the battle.

"I was always a fierce admirer of Abraham Lincoln, and his vision of what was 'suffered and done' at Gettysburg captured my imagination at an early age," Doug will tell anyone who listens. "I love the story of the nation as it is told at Gettysburg… stories of the soldiers, the citizens, the leader and the choices they made, the history they shaped, and the nation they forged."

While a strong Christian, husband, father, and proud Marine Corps officer, Doug also recently passed the extremely difficult test associated with becoming a licensed battlefield guide. He, his wife, and two sons live in a Civil War house on Seminary Ridge, across which General Longstreet marched his soldiers on the second day of the battle.

Colonel Douds's support proved to be indispensable to the learning and success we would achieve in only one day.

The Battle

It would be nearly impossible, as well as wholly unnecessary, to summarize the Battle of Gettysburg for the purposes of this book. Anyway, we wanted to use the events of the three days, and the personalities of those involved, as a vehicle for discussing leadership.

We arrived by charter flight the night before the ride. Early the next morning, while our participants ate breakfast in the hotel dining room, Colonel Douds gave the group a strategic overview. He discussed the political issues affecting both President Lincoln and President Davis and the campaigns raging in the other theaters of the war, Kentucky/ Tennessee and Vicksburg (in the latter, General Grant would declare victory the same day the Gettysburg Battle concluded), which would affect what happened in Pennsylvania. Then he discussed the movement of both Southern and Northern forces from their previous positions near Chancellorsville, Virginia, and how that movement affected the timeline of the Gettysburg campaign. He showed the group the weapons used and the logistics employed, and he described the education and training of the soldiers and officers who fought one another.

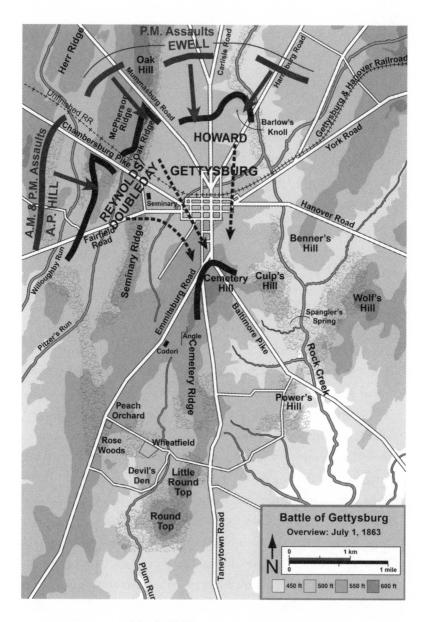

Map by Hal Jepersen, www.cwmaps.com

Then we boarded buses that moved us to the first of ten "stands" where we would learn about and describe important pieces of the battle.

The first day of the battle, July 1, featured a "meeting engagement," basically a collision of two armies to the northwest and north of the town of Gettysburg. A Union cavalry division under Cavalryman Brigadier General John Buford, reinforced with two Union corps throughout the morning and early afternoon, defended ridges, tree lines, and creeks to the northwest of town. Early in the morning, two large Confederate corps began an assault from the northwest, and then an additional corps added to the fight later in the day. All of this created a desperate fight and sent the Union defenders retreating through the town to the hills overlooking Gettysburg.

The fighting grew more intense as the day wore on. It is sometimes said the Southerners needed either to win early or get repulsed all day to gain a victory, but neither of these things happened. We stopped at four locations to discuss the first day of the fight, commenting on such subjects as traits of a leader, building consensus while understanding the motivations of others, and the use of initiative and trust.

On the second day of battle, both armies assembled in either offensive or defensive positions around the town. The Union positions were laid out in a defensive formation resembling a fishhook, while the Confederates still mustered forces from several directions all around western Pennsylvania. While initially he did not want to order an assault, Lee finally decided—against the advice of many of his subordinates, who did not effectively "lead up"—to attack the Union left flank on the late afternoon of July 2. Fierce fighting raged at the Peach Orchard, the Wheatfield, Devil's Den, and Little Round Top. All across the battlefield, despite significant losses and continued movement into new positions, Union defenders held the line.

Again, we moved the class to various stands where we discussed how the enemy gets a vote whenever leaders come together, how personalities matter in leader-led relationships, and how leaders must understand what their organization is attempting to accomplish so they can contribute to its success.

On July 3, fighting resumed on Culp's Hill while cavalry battles raged to the east and south, but the main event involved a dramatic infantry assault by 12,500 Confederates against the center of the Union line

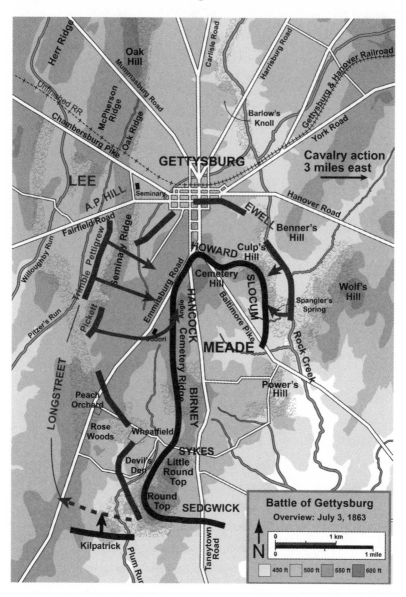

Map by Hal Jepersen, www.cwmaps.com

(known officially as the Pickett-Pettigrew Assault, but which has gained fame as "Pickett's Charge"). Our physician leaders walked this deadly space that became hallowed ground, and they marveled at the stories Colonel Douds told along the way about the sacrifice and dedication of those who selflessly gave their last full measure in a ludicrous attempt to achieve a victory. The discussion centered on confidence and arrogance, understanding subordinates, and dedication to the profession.

What We Learned

As we came to each stand, Colonel Douds asked various individuals to tell the group about "their" battlefield character. They did so in the first person ("Hello, my name is General Lee… let me tell you some things about myself and my plan"), and most of them provided a bit of flair and panache to their stories. As they viewed the land where more than 150 years before their historical counterpart had stood and made tough leadership decisions, they had to respond to a simple question: "What are you thinking?"

Since the physician leaders now saw history and the requirements for leadership in a different light than they had only months before, they had to describe "their" decisions in a pragmatic way. It went something like this:

> **A doctor**: *My character was General Meade. When I read he was promoted to be the commanding general of the Union Forces just three days before the battle, after General Hooker was relieved, it seemed incomprehensible that someone would ask him to do that. He was given so much authority and responsibility on the eve of a very important event.*
>
> *But when he took command, he used a consensus building*

approach to influence his subordinates, a technique we have discussed in class. He realized that some knew more than he did and were probably better field commanders, so he asked them to contribute to the plan and the execution. Then, after they came up with a plan, he delegated responsibility. He spent a lot of time riding around the battlefield, ensuring his subordinates were doing what he had told them to do and that they were contributing to what he wanted to accomplish. It was obvious he was developing trust with them, and as the days wore on, they started achieving victory for the first time against the Confederates.

It hit me that someday all of us are going to be asked to fill leadership positions in the hospital. Instead of saying, "Holy smokes. Am I ready for this? Do I have the right skills?" I can do some analysis. Get feedback from others. Go to those who have the information, who have the experience, to see if they can provide ideas that might help before I go off on a tirade. It's a lot better approach than believing you have all the answers when you're new to a position, when it's really likely that won't be the case.

A nurse: *I had General Sickles as my character, and it seemed to me he was really insecure about who he was—he was a politician among a group of West Pointers who knew how to soldier—and he didn't quite understand what he was being asked to do. He did the best he could, but he didn't make the right decisions, and his actions caused a lot of his people to die and almost caused a break in the line.*

It hit me that all leaders are insecure, to some degree. That's probably not something we think about. But what might affect you as a leader is the level of insecurity you exhibit and knowing that the speed at which you overcome it is what separates the not so good from the great leaders.

A doctor: *I played Colonel Chamberlain. Here's this guy who is a college professor before the war starts, he doesn't know anything about soldiering, and now he's in a critical position where he has to lead his soldiers and make tough decisions. It struck me that he admitted to himself he didn't know everything, but he was constantly trying to learn new things about his role, about tactics, and about his people. He realized his people wanted him to succeed because of the person he was... they wanted to be associated with him because of his values, his attributes, how he cared for them, and how he was focused on the mission. And they just liked being around him. He had the right approach in a new position, and he brought the team in. He showed them he was genuine, he had the right vision for the organization, and he communicated that vision continuously.*

An administrator: *I was General Lee. For me, I learned two things that I realize I can apply in my hospital.*

First, it's great to have a good strategic vision of where you want to take the organization, but if you don't continuously communicate that vision and get feedback on where you stand— with your people and with your superiors—then it really won't matter.

Second, the importance of creating a sense of ownership on what you want as an end result of any endeavor is critical. Lee came to Pennsylvania on the premise of accomplishing something, but then he didn't listen to Longstreet and his other commanders when they told him he was going off track and doing something completely different. This battle is an example of the Confederate Army failing on the vision and the communication, and the Union Army succeeding by using those same two things to their advantage.

I didn't realize how those parts of leadership can be so difficult, because you have to continuously assess your vision to see if you're still going in the right direction. And you have to continuously communicate what you're trying to accomplish to those around you… and yourself.

A doctor*: I was Dr. Letterman, and I had to take care of all the wounded on the battlefield. One of the things I realized is that whether you're in war or in healthcare, a willingness to take chances and work with administrators or generals who are willing to take those same chances is very important. I don't want people not to try something because they're afraid to make a mistake. But you still have to recognize you're being graded on being willing to try to change a process.*

We did some different things in treating our wounded at Gettysburg, and that was because we had the blessing of the generals to try something new.

A doctor*: My character was General Heth, and I really screwed up the first day for General Lee because I didn't do what he told me to do. I didn't believe the enemy in front of me was all that tough.*

It really struck me when Colonel Douds kept repeating that the enemy gets a vote. I didn't understand it at first, but then I started thinking: We don't necessarily have enemies in healthcare, but we do have a lot of moving parts and different agendas. I think anytime you decide that you're going to implement a strategy or plan, you have to realize it's not in a static model; more likely, there are going to be reactions from different groups who may not like what you're doing. You're going to have to address those people and their concerns or they will continue to be a thorn in your side, just like Buford's cavalry was to me.

A doctor: *I was General Lee. As we walked across Pickett's Charge, Colonel Douds asked me, "So, General Lee, how are you doing? Give me an assessment… not from what you know happens at the end, but what you know right now as the attack is proceeding."*

I said, "I'm not sure right now, but I don't think we're doing very well. We may penetrate the middle and the men are still charging, but we have no reinforcements and I didn't think about that before I sent these guys in."

That exchange really affected me, as I realized that we must make constant assessments as a leader. We can't just wait until things are all over to do it, because then it may be too late. It seems to me that sometimes when we say we want to do something, as a leader, we need a plan to assess things as they are taking place. As leaders, we need to continuously reevaluate.

And then I realized I didn't give permission for others to "lead up" to me. I learned from General Lee's mistake that no matter how good you are, you must listen to your subordinates and assess what they say. You may be 4-0-1, as Lee was before Gettysburg, but no matter how good you have been in the past, you should still trust those around you to help you with your decision making. As a leader, you should help establish a cadre of people who can speak truth to power. Lee had that with Longstreet, but for some reason, he didn't listen to his trusted advisors at a critical time. That's especially important as a doctor, because a lot of people treat us like God, and I'm not sure we give permission to others to speak the truth to us. We need to do a better job of that.

A nurse: *I was General Ewell, and I was new to command. The two common themes that are elements of success came down to knowing your situation and your people. Those who failed* *misunderstood one or the other.*

General Lee was very successful, but he had a bunch of new people like me as his subordinates that he didn't understand, and he didn't communicate very well with them. Meade, on the other hand, understood the situation and found a way to understand his people. You have to get both right; you can't get one or the other right.

A doctor*: I was General Jeb Stuart, one of Lee's trusted advisors who failed him. We were taught that trust is key, and trusted advisors are even more important. It was very interesting, his lack of flexibility, particularly in regards to Stuart… He didn't send out his other cavalrymen to do the job that needed to be done. That, to me, was a revelation. I was completely unaware of that, and that's a big deal.*

A doctor*: I had an interesting character, General Hancock. He was probably the smartest and the most capable general on either side. But he didn't flaunt it. He was humble. He built trust with the others and helped them succeed.*

As I listened to others speak throughout the day, the element of trust with their subordinates and their superiors seemed to separate the losers from the winners. After all we've talked about regarding attributes and competencies, and leading down and leading up and building teams, it hit me that leaders do one thing: they develop trust within an organization. People trust leaders to do the right things. They trust you to look out for their welfare. They trust you to advance and win on the battlefield, or they trust you to fix the things related to healthcare. If you're arrogant and you haven't generated that trust among the people you're working with, down, up, and sideways, you're probably not much of a leader.

After spending an amazing day on a Civil War battlefield, the importance and the application of critical leadership lessons got driven home in a unique and powerful way. But the real test of learning came not in a national park, but in the hospital trenches back home.

Leaders Changing Healthcare

Within weeks of completing the PLD course, all of our inaugural graduates got asked to serve in both formal and informal positions. One physician got invited to serve as the chief medical officer of our children's hospital. Another was asked to become the medical director of our new women's hospital. Many received invitations to serve on committees for the Clinical Integrated Network (CIN), where they will lead various initiatives destined to change the shape of healthcare in Central Florida.

We watched as our graduates gathered together to lead change with well-thought-out and analytical approaches, engaging with others in professional dialogue, and building teams tasked with addressing key issues.

Jay asked for help with a destination medicine project in India, and every physician of Indian descent in the class contributed. One clinician, who was also studying for a PhD, came to us with a request for help with her thesis proposal. She wanted to show that the HCAHPS and Patient Engagement scores would get a bump because of the training received by those who had attended the course. Her gut told her it would be evident, based on the changes she already had seen in the physicians, but she wanted to prove it—the first of many research projects on the value of the Physician Development Leadership Class.

WAR STORY

From "Before" to "After"

A graduate of our PLD course recently accompanied Jay and me on a trip to Nigeria. Since he was familiar with the way we used war stories, I asked him to write one about his own leadership journey.

So there I was…

The slipstream rushing over the fuselage whirled along with my rising excitement over the adventure ahead. Then I finally felt the subtle reduction in power the pilot applied to the turbines, followed by the much-anticipated slow descending arc toward our destination. We were about to land. I closed my notebook and craned my neck for that coveted first glimpse of the African continent.

Sitting next to me, General Hertling had just enjoyed his last good meal for the week. A grin lingered at the corners of his mouth. At six four, the man had a commanding view of the cabin—and I had seen him glancing at my travel diary. I feared an idea had taken root.

"Are you writing bad things about me?" he joked.

As I contemplated how to remain relevant to the task of forging an international business relationship between the largest hospital in Florida and an Adventist university in Nigeria, the general smiled and leaned in.

"Joe… I have a mission for you," he said.

My aggressive optimism and overwillingness to participate had become a punch line by this point in the trip. I belted out, "This is an excellent mission, sir. I am happy to help in any way, sir!"

The general and I shared another laugh. How in the world did *I* get myself picked to be *here*? Without a hitch, he led me back on track.

"I want you to keep track of moments in this trip," he said, pointing at my notebook. "Note whenever you feel as if you handle things differently than you would have before you took the leadership course. Your practical thoughts would help me make the course more valuable if I knew exactly how you benefit from what we do in there."

A short while later, my hair matted with sweat, I stood in a dimly lit Nigerian customs area. A man slung with an exceptionally high mileage Kalashnikov was arguing with me over the validity of my yellow fever vaccination. He was adamant that the bright yellow vaccination card was undated. The card was clearly dated. My inner smart mouth squirmed.

"Thank you for taking the time to review my records," I said instead. "I know you're working hard." The man waived me through the line as though I had performed the Jedi mind trick on him. The old me would have ended up detained.

And so the adventure commenced.

My journey to Africa by way of a much-needed self-improvement program had begun a year and a half before. I was on the verge of either quitting or getting fired from my practice. I had passed burnout so long ago that I felt nostalgic for being merely dissatisfied in my work. Though I served on numerous hospital committees, no one would listen to me. The world, it seemed to me, kept spinning more and more out of control.

Standing in a busy hospital hallway, I was arguing on the phone with my partner when a representative from the PLD approached. My administrative friends had "strongly encouraged" me to sign up for the classes, and I had done so. Without ending my call, I took the twenty-pound bag of books and grimaced at the woman who had delivered them. Though I indeed read every page of those books, my initial impressions were (predictably) bleak.

The first session hit me like a belt sander. General Hertling, whom I had never met, introduced himself and his colleague, Colonel Jay Voorhees, to a suspicious crowd of doctors burdened with feelings similar to my own. In his opening remarks, he revealed that he had been roaming the hospital incognito for weeks, observing the class members in their day-to-day lives. To cite an example of how abrasive some members of the medical staff could be, he quoted "one young doctor" as having accused an entire department of "taking good people and making them stupid."

Oh great, I thought as I felt the blood rush into my cheeks. *That was me*. I was the poster boy for "before."

Desperate to stay in the game, I threw up my hand. "What would you consider to be a successful outcome for this class on leadership?" I asked the general, with probably more than a hint of sarcasm. Mark bit his lower lip and pointed at me. Sixty people looked at me, to General Hertling, and back to me.

"I want to light *your* fire," he answered slowly.

He launched into a long overview of the class, filled with information about "leadership" and "professionalism" and the like. We ended the day with a uniformly depressing dive into our personality assessment results. More than once, I read words like "caustic" and "scary" on my own results. At that moment, I realized I didn't like who I had let myself become. I didn't even understand that I was responsible for the way people saw me, but I knew I didn't want to be feared and avoided any longer. Something deep inside me took the general's spark.

Over the next year, I devoted myself to a heightened sense of personal awareness. Whenever I interacted with anyone, I tried to remain

conscious of how my words and actions might impact them. Whenever
I encountered a situation where I might be required to correct or redirect
someone, I made diligent efforts to do so in a constructive manner.

People noticed.

I came to understand that I had not always made my intentions clear
and that I didn't always project a professional and respectful bearing.
I changed by adopting rules designed to respect those with whom I work.
A once devoted scrubs-and-sneakers man, I began to wear a jacket and
tie to meetings. I realized that I had not set a good example for my staff
and patients, so I began to exercise regularly and eat a healthy diet. I
fought my natural tendency toward sarcasm and levity while trying to
replace those characteristics with optimism and humility.

Slowly, but surely, I found myself not only involved in, but immersed
in, project after project with my hospital system. I was elected chairman
of the department of medicine, and from that new post I have been able
to effectively engage administration and medical staff to effect changes
I truly believe benefit patients, doctors, and the hospital system alike. I
mended fences with my colleagues and have once again become a bedrock
partner of our growing fifty-doctor practice.

When my leadership mentors, Mark and Jay, asked me if I would have
any interest in traveling with them as they conducted some international
work, I couldn't believe that of all the doctors present on that first day of
leadership training, they now thought of me as an ambassador for the
hospital. I felt that not only had I been the poster-boy for "before," I was
now a legitimate contender for the "after," as well.

In our visit to Nigeria, I saw the best and worst of what leadership
can be. I saw how great leaders can change the very idea of what is possible and elevate a nation. I saw how toxic leadership can leave an entire
people bereft of hope. In four of the most whirlwind days of my life, I
saw most clearly how I had changed as a leader. I realized that without
accepting the changes I needed to make, not only would I have failed
in my career, but I would also have become unhappy in life. Working

with Mark and Jay in Nigeria—through maddening, even dangerous challenges—I finally came to fully appreciate how much these two men had helped me.

When we finally started making our way home (a string of canceled flights awaited us), I jotted down the lessons that became clear to me in our travels. I hope you will find these simple lessons effective in bettering your own relationships. After all, relationships are the backbone of all we do. I would stress the following insights to any leader:

1. *Be On Time. If you are late, you will hinder progress, frustrate those who are on time, and appear to be disorganized and disrespectful of those with whom you work.*

2. *Actively Cooperate. Always seek mutually beneficial opportunities to drive productivity by remaining involved in overcoming barriers.*

3. *Humility Invites Kindness. Let your effectiveness and respect for others speak to your greatness. Courtesy and generosity will determine your treatment.*

4. *Optimism Invites Trust. No one seeks to forge negative relationships. If you truly work to remain positive, others will place their trust in your desire to do good.*

5. *Trust Is the Gateway to Opportunity. If you do not trust your organization or colleagues, ask yourself what your values really are and why you are doing what you are doing.*

6. *Be Concise. Your words will be more powerful if you choose them carefully.*

7. *Familiarity Is Superior to Formality. Be human, be honest, be open.*

*You will find people make themselves more available to you if they see
you for who you really are (and many of them will like you, anyway).*

DR. CHRISTOPHER "JOE" SMITH
Chairman of Medicine
AdventHealth, Orlando, Florida
Assistant Professor of Clinical Medicine
Florida State University/University of Central Florida

Epilogue

The Anonymous Letter

Ashort while after we finished our inaugural Physician Leadership Development course, an anonymous letter arrived in my office. The unidentified writer had signed it, "one of your PLD students." Have you ever received an anonymous letter? Usually, you duck for cover to stay safe from flying shrapnel. So I sat down, took a deep breath, opened the letter, and steeled myself for the worst.

I did not at all expect what I found. But allow me to let him/her tell his/her own story:

My first thought before beginning the course was, "It's nice the hospital appears to be concerned about physician leadership, but is this going to be another gesture without any real meaning?" What made me apply was that I wanted to help move things along, and I thought I might be able to learn from a couple of army guys.

When we began our monthly meetings, I was struck by what appeared to be a combination of skepticism, frustration, but also a willingness to listen and learn on the part of the members of the class. This was something new. What I saw were a number of people who, like me, had spent a great deal of time and effort trying to be helpful and generally desiring to work with the hospital, but they just wouldn't listen to us! There were a lot of people who seemed to be tired of beating their heads against the wall when they knew there was a better solution.

As we progressed through the course, what I realized was that much of the frustration was due to not knowing how to communicate... not knowing how to speak the language of those we were dealing with. I think we also all started to realize and understand what would be the system-wide ramifications of seemingly small and inconsequential suggestions we were making. I also learned that a "seat at the table," which we all wanted, required some table manners, which few of us had.

I think the biggest thing I will take away from this course—besides the great friendships, the bonds between different kinds of healthcare professionals, and an understanding of things about leadership that I never knew before—is that, as physicians, the future of healthcare is in our hands, but only if we take an active role in shaping that future. Change is coming to a healthcare system that cannot possibly survive in its current state, and no amount of stubbornness or complaining by a bunch of doctors will prevent that. If we as physicians continue to fight a battle that already has been decided, then someone else will decide our future.

In attending the Physician Leadership Course, I realized that the nucleus for change is present; as a result of this course, we have a ready-made group of professionals (and I now understand that word much better) who have the skill set to begin the difficult task of shaping our healthcare future. And I now also know we have an influential partner in AdventHealth to assist us in this challenge. Whether we are up to the task is completely up to each of us.

Since the end of the class, I've had a number of opportunities. While I still have occasional challenges when dealing with specific people or with specific projects, I know I am now better prepared to use the skills I learned in the course. And my values are pointing the way. Thanks for all you've done to help me on my journey.

I've received a lot of letters in my career, and more than a few of them from a cranky Mr. or Ms. Anonymous. It's nice to get one without any shrapnel at all.

ACKNOWLEDGMENTS

I once heard that there are no coincidences, only events where God wishes to remain anonymous. Our chief medical officer, Dr. Dave Moorhead, our chief clinical officer, Sheryl Dodds, and our chief operating officer, Brian Paradis, had wanted to "do something different to develop physician leaders" for several years. While some may think it serendipitous that an old, retired general arrived at an opportune time to provide some thoughts on how we might do that, I think it was a blessing for all of us. I learned an awful lot about healthcare and how doctors view life, and hopefully they learned that physicians have talents that can create miracles beyond healing. I am proud to be a member of their team, and the "command climate" they've fostered is phenomenal.

Colonel (retired) Jay Voorhees helped design the innovative Physician Leader Course, and then assisted in birthing it with masterful class commentary and brilliant mentoring of our healthcare professionals. Jay is blessed with a charismatic style, an ever-present smile, and a desire to help others grow in leadership skills; he is the perfect teammate, trainer... and friend. We were both assisted in getting the *right* healthcare professionals into the course by Ms. Lee Johnson, who is the director of Physician Strategic Development, Dr. Moorhead's trusted deputy, and the "mother" for all the doctors at AdventHealth Orlando. Lee is a wonderful, giving person, and she gave both Jay and me continuous advice and assistance, and helped make the course so successful. Helping all stay on track (and providing comic relief along the way) was a stable of assistants—Liliana Parra, Daisy Lopez, and Ivelisse Alexandrou—who ensured our doctors received CME credits for the classes, took attendance, arranged for food, and delivered books; they are a unique group of professionals, and we are blessed to have them working with us.

There were several doctors in our first Physician Leader Course who so enjoyed our journey they suggested a book to describe the experience. Todd Chobotar, our director of AdventHealth Press, thought that a fascinating idea. Always more than a supporter, Todd continuously provided sage guidance on how we might best approach a project that would both describe how we were changing our environment and how others might do the same. I owe him a great deal of gratitude for helping interpret the vision for this book. But I also owe him for introducing me to Steve Halliday, our book "polisher." He took a crude first draft, made terrific suggestions, hosted me for a final weekend of crafting, and the result is this product, which he also now believes might contribute to the improved health of our nation.

When I was a child, the old bookmobile would come to our parochial school, and by happenstance I picked up a book entitled *West Point Plebe*, written by Red Reeder. That book, and the others in the Clint Lane series, inspired me to want to go to the Military Academy. I later found out that Red Reeder was quite a character, but also a war hero with a distinguished and fascinating career. But his active career ended when he was leading his regiment and lost his leg on Normandy's Utah Beach. General Omar Bradley sent him home to recover at West Point, and he became quite a fixture at the academy, eventually becoming the athletic director during the heyday of army sports. He wrote myriad books about the academy, military life, and the philosophies of soldiering, and he is buried at West Point, next to the Cadet Chapel. His tombstone reads, in part, "Colonel Russell 'Red' Reeder: Soldier, Coach, Author." Next to Red is the grave of his wife, Dorothea, who all the cadets knew as "Ms. Dort." On her grave is a simpler epithet: "Dorothea Reeder, Red's Editor."

My terrific wife, Sue, is my Dorothea Reeder. She left her home in New York to follow me all over the world, always made our government quarters into a warm and cozy home, and most importantly, she "loves her soldier, proudly." Sue gives me daily inspiration with her grace and style, and she wears a velvet glove when providing tough critiques. More than anyone, she helped me with this book... and she constantly gives me a purpose for life.

NOTES

1. WHO, *World Health Statistics* 2011 (Geneva: World Health Organization, 2011), ISBN 978-92-4-156419-9.

2. Sean Keehan, Andrea Sisko, Christopher Truffer, Sheila Smith, Cathy Cowan, John Poisal, M. Kent Clemens, and the National Health Expenditure Accounts Projections Team, "Health Spending Projections Through 2017: The Baby-Boom Generation Is Coming To Medicare," *Health Affairs* 27, no. 2 (March 2008): w145–w155, Web Exclusive, February 26, 2008, retrieved February 27, 2008, doi: 10.1377/hlthaff.27.2.w145.

3. Dinah Walker, "Trends in US Defense Military Spending," Council on Foreign Relations Report, July 15, 2014.

4. Falcone, BE and B Satiani (2008), "Physician as Hospital Chief Executive Officer," *Vascular and Endovascular Surgery* 42, no. 1 (February/March 2008): 88–94, doi: 10.1177/1538574407309320.

5. The PLD program we designed for AdventHealth extensively uses elements from the leadership model found in ADRP 6-22.

6. A variety of excellent works discuss professions and professional behavior. See Larson's *The Rise of Professionalism: A Sociological Analysis* (1978); Jackson's *Professions and Professionalization* (2010); and Montgomery's *Medicine, Accountability, and Professionalism* (1989). My favorite, *The Future of the Army Profession*, is a compendium of articles discussing professional elements and behaviors, edited by Don M. Snider and published in 2005.

7. This definition, taken from chapter 2 of *The Future of the Army Profession*, describes the "expertise, jurisdiction, and legitimacy" of the military profession.

8. Hamilton, JS, "Scribonius Largus on the Medical Profession," *Bulletin of the History of Medicine* 60 (1986): 209–16.

9. Edelstein, L., *The Hippocratic Oath: Text, Translation and Interpretation* (Baltimore, MD: Johns Hopkins University Press, 1943).

10. The Alpha Omega Alpha Honor Medical Society has been particularly active in discussing professionalism and professional behavior. Its 2015 monograph, "Medical Professionalism: Best Practices," edited by Drs. Richard Byyny, Maxine Papadakis, and Douglas Paauw is a masterful attempt at discussing the elements of the modern medical profession.

11. The basic concept of leader attributes and competencies comes from ADRP 6-22, although we've adapted some words to better fit the requirements of physician leaders.

12. Most senior military leaders refer to a great book titled *Generalship: Its Diseases and Their Cure*, by J.F.C. Fuller.

13. Most of these "methods of influence" are taken from the army's leadership manual ADRP 6-22; the examples used in the explanations are my own attempt to provide connection between the military and healthcare.

14. KJ Swayden, KK Anderson, LM Connelly, JS Moran, JK McMahon, PM Arnold, "Effect of Sitting vs. Standing on Perception of Provider Time at Bedside: A Pilot Study," *Patient Education and Counseling* 86, no. 2 (Feb. 2012):166–71, doi: 10.1016/j.pec.2011.05.024, accessed online via PubMed on 08-10-15, http://www.ncbi.nlm.nih.gov/pubmed/21719234.

15. I feel extremely fortunate to have been allowed to fund and conduct battle staff rides at every level of command. I have experienced unit staff rides to Gettysburg, Shiloh, Antietam, Little Big Horn, Vicksburg, and others in the US; Normandy, St Lô, Anzio, Bastogne, Huertgen Forest, Ardennes, and others in Europe; Kiev, Warsaw, and St. Petersburg in Ukraine, Poland, and Russia; and even Gaugamela—the fight between Alexander the Great and Darius—on the Ninevah Plains of Iraq. That last battlefield was the most interesting, as we brought along some of our Iraqi Army counterparts to experience this event, and it was the only staff ride that I've had interrupted by a firefight with insurgents.

About the Author

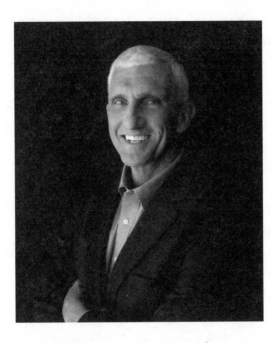

General Mark Hertling retired in 2013 after serving almost four decades in the US Army. After retiring from the Army, Hertling became a senior vice president at AdventHealth Orlando, with a portfolio addressing global partnering, health programs for employees and the community, and leadership development for physicians and executives.

Immediately before retiring from the Army, Mark commanded US Army Europe and Seventh Army where he led over forty thousand soldiers, cared for over one hundred thousand family members, and partnered with the militaries and governments of fifty countries in Europe.

During his military career, LTG Hertling commanded units at every level, from a 19-soldier tank platoon to a 90,000 multinational task force. While in the military, Hertling was known as a soldier-focused trainer, a savvy operator, a strategic visionary, and an expert in multinational engagements.

Hertling holds a Bachelor of Science degree from the US Military Academy at West Point, and is a graduate of the Army's Staff College, the School of Advanced Military Studies, and the National War College. He holds Master of Arts Degrees in Military Art and Science and International Relations and Security Studies from the Army's Staff College and the National War College, and a Master of Science in Exercise Physiology from Indiana University. In 2019, he defended a dissertation addressing leadership in healthcare at the Crummer School of Business at Rollins College, and was awarded a Doctor of Business Administration from that institution.

Hertling holds numerous military awards, including the Distinguished Service Medal, the Legion of Merit, the Bronze Stars, and the Purple Heart. He has also received awards from the governments of Germany, Poland, Romania, Saudi Arabia, and Kuwait. He received the Dwight Eisenhower Award from the US Sports Academy, and in 2019 he received the Indiana University School of Health Science Distinguished Alumni Award.

In retirement, Mark was appointed by President Obama to be one of twenty-five members of the President's Council on Fitness, Sports and Nutrition, where he served from 2013-2017. Hertling serves as a military analyst for CNN, and he speaks and acts passionately on the subjects of leadership, national security, and health trends.

Mark is married to his best friend, Sue. They have two married sons and four grandchildren. He loves being with family, reading history, bicycling, and any form of athletic activity.

ABOUT THE PUBLISHER

AdventHealth is a connected network of care that promotes hope and healing through individualized care that touches the body, mind and spirit to help you feel whole. Our hospitals and care sites across the country are united by one mission: Extending the Healing Ministry of Christ. This faith-based mission guides our skilled and compassionate caregivers to provide expert care that leads the nation in quality, safety, and patient satisfaction.

Over 5 million people visit AdventHealth each year at our award-winning hospitals, physician practices, outpatient clinics, skilled nursing facilities, home health agencies and hospice centers to experience wholistic care for any stage of life and health.

AdventHealth Press publishes content rooted in wholistic health principles to help you feel whole through a variety of physical, emotional, and spiritual wellness resources. To learn more visit **AdventHealthPress.com**.

RECOGNITIONS

CLINICAL EXCELLENCE. AdventHealth hospital campuses have been recognized in the top five percent of hospitals in the nation for clinical excellence by Healthgrades. We believe that spiritual and emotional care, along with high-quality clinical care, combine to create the best outcome for our patients.

TOP SAFETY RATINGS. We care for you like we would care for our own loved ones — with compassion and a priority of safety. AdventHealth's hospitals have received grade "A" safety ratings from The Leapfrog Group, the only national rating agency that evaluates how well hospitals protect patients from medical errors, infections, accidents, and injuries.

SPECIALIZED CARE. For over ten years, AdventHealth hospitals have been recognized by U.S. News & World Report as "One of America's Best Hospitals" for clinical specialties such as: Cardiology and Heart Surgery, Orthopedics, Neurology and Neuroscience, Urology, Gynecology, Gastroenterology and GI Surgery, Diabetes and Endocrinology, Pulmonology, Nephrology, and Geriatrics.

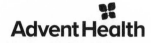

AWARD-WINNING TEAM CULTURE. Becker's Hospital Review has recognized AdventHealth as a Top Place to Work in Healthcare based on diversity, team engagement and professional growth. AdventHealth has also been awarded for fostering an engaged workforce, meaning our teams are equipped and empowered in their work as they provide skilled and compassionate care.

PARTNERSHIPS

WALT DISNEY WORLD. AdventHealth has teamed up with the Walt Disney World® Resort to serve as the health and wellness resource partner that cares for cast members and guests from around the world. Disney and AdventHealth partnered to create a state-of-the-art children's hospital and a cutting-edge comprehensive health facility that was named the "Hospital of the Future" by the Wall Street Journal.

SPORTS TEAMS. AdventHealth is the official hospital for the NBA's Orlando Magic, NFL's Tampa Bay Buccaneers, NHL's Tampa Bay Lightning, the Orlando Solar Bears, The University of Central Florida Knights, RunDisney, and sponsor of Daytona Speedweeks (NASCAR). In addition, AdventHealth has served as the exclusive medical care provider to many sports organizations such as Disney's Wide World of Sports, Walt Disney World's Marathon Weekend, the Capital One Bowl, and University of Central Florida Athletics. AdventHealth has also provided comprehensive healthcare services for the World Cup and the Olympics.

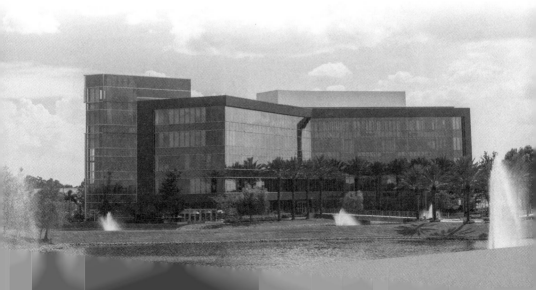

LEAD YOUR COMMUNITY
TO HEALTHY
LIVING

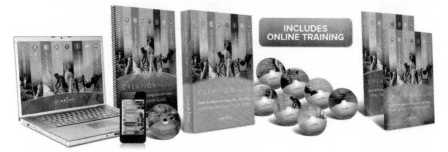
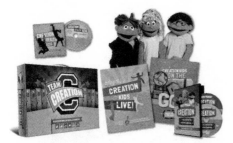
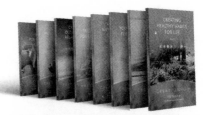

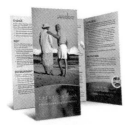

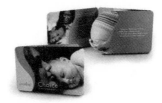

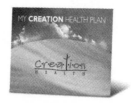

Senior Guide
Share the CREATION Life principles with seniors and help them be healthier and happier as they live life to the fullest.

Pregnancy Guides
Expert advice on how to experience CREATION Life while expecting.

Pocket Guide
A tool for keeping people committed to living all of the CREATION Life principles daily.

Tote Bag
A convenient way for bringing CREATION Life materials to and from class.

Tumbler
Practice good Nutrition and keep yourself hydrated with a CREATION Life tumbler in an assortment of fun colors.

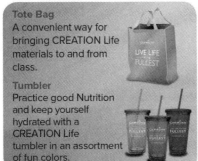

MARKETING MATERIALS

Postcards, Posters, Stationery, and More
You can effectively advertise and generate community excitement about your CREATION Life seminar with a wide range of available marketing materials such as enticing postcards, flyers, posters, and more.

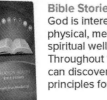

Bible Stories
God is interested in our physical, mental and spiritual well-being. Throughout the Bible you can discover the eight principles for full life.

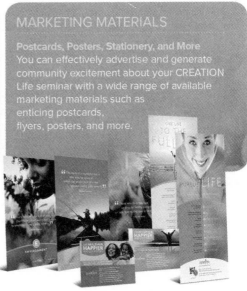

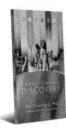

CREATION Life Discovery
Written by Des Cummings Jr., PhD, Monica Reed, MD, and Todd Chobotar, this wonderful resource introduces people to the CREATION Life philosophy and lifestyle.

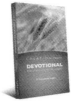

CREATION Life Devotional
(English: Hardcover / Spanish: Softcover) In this devotional you will discover stories about experiencing God's grace in the tough times, God's delight in triumphant times, and God's presence in peaceful times.

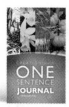

CREATION Life One-Sentence Journal

The *CREATION Life One-Sentence Journal* is a simple, fun, and powerful tool to transform your life. It takes just moments a day, yet the effect it can have over time is life-changing.

CREATION Life Devotional for Women

Written for women by women, the CREATION Life Devotional for Women is based on the principles of whole-person wellness represented in CREATION Life. Spirits will be lifted and lives rejuvenated by the message of each unique chapter.

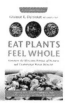

CREATION Health Breakthrough

Blending science and lifestyle recommendations, Monica Reed, MD, prescribes eight essentials that will help reverse harmful health habits and prevent disease. Discover how intentional choices, rest, environment, activity, trust, relationships, outlook, and nutrition can put a person on the road to wellness.

Scalpel Moments

A scalpel moment can be one of painful awareness, disturbing clarity, sorrowful regret. It can also be a moment of positive awakening that can reveal, restore, and renew. Ordained minister Dr. Reaves highlights stories about life's difficult or revealing moments that remove layers of confusion, bitterness, or fear and restore one's trust in God.

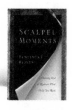

Eat Plants Feel Whole

For over thirty years, Dr. Guthrie has been helping his patients gain better health through an evidence-based, whole-food, plant-based lifestyle. Now, in *Eat Plants, Feel Whole*, he shares not only his years of expertise with you, but the scientific evidence to back it up as well.

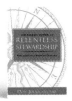

The Hidden Power of Relentless Stewardship

Dr. Jernigan shows how an organization's culture can be molded to create high performance at every level, fulfilling mission and vision, while wisely utilizing —or stewarding — the limited resources of time, money, and energy.

Leadership in the Crucible of Work

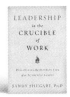

What is the first and most important work of a leader? (The answer may surprise you.) In *Leadership in the Crucible of Work*, noted speaker, poet, and college president Dr. Sandy Shugart takes readers on an unforgettable journey to the heart of what it means to become an authentic leader.

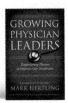

Growing Physician Leaders

Retired Army Lieutenant General Mark Hertling applies his four decades of military leadership to the work of healthcare, resulting in a profoundly constructive and practical book with the power to reshape and re-energize any healthcare organization in America today.

Health and Healing Bible Promises

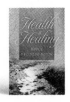

The Bible is packed with promises on health and healing - from aging to nutrition to rest, from grief to anger to stress. The *Health and Healing Bible Promises* book collects over 600 scriptures in more than thirty different translations in a convenient pocket size on these topics and more including the CREATION Life principles.

The Love Fight

Are you going to fight for love or against each other? The authors illustrate how this common encounter can create a mutually satisfying relationship. Their expertise will walk you through the scrimmage between those who want to accomplish and those who want to relate.

AdventHealthPress.com

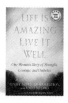

Life Is Amazing Live It Well

At its heart, Linda's captivating account chronicles the struggle to reconcile her three dreams of experiencing life as a "normal woman" with the tough realities of her medical condition. Her journey is punctuated with insights that are at times humorous, painful, provocative, and life-affirming.

Pain Free For Life

In *Pain Free For Life*, Scott C. Brady, MD,—founder of Florida Hospital's Brady Institute for Health—leads pain-racked readers to a pain-free life using powerful mind-body-spirit strategies—where more than 80 percent of his chronic-pain patients have achieved 80–100 percent pain relief within weeks.

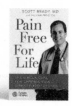

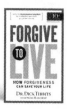

Forgive To Live (English: Hardcover/Spanish: Softcover)

In *Forgive To Live: How Forgiveness Can Save Your Life*, Dr. Tibbits presents the scientifically proven steps for forgiveness—taken from the first clinical study of its kind conducted by Stanford University and Florida Hospital.

Forgive To Live Devotional

In his powerful new devotional Dr. Dick Tibbits reveals the secret to forgiveness. This compassionate devotional is a stirring look at the true meaning of forgiveness. Each of the 56 spiritual insights includes motivational Scripture, an inspirational prayer, and two thought-provoking questions. The insights are designed to encourage your journey as you begin to *Forgive to Live*.

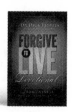

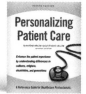

Personalizing Patient Care

Personalizing Patient Care is a valuable guide for improving a caregiver's understanding of how a patient's background may affect their needs, preferences, and expectations related to the delivery of care. This unique, field-tested reference will enable healthcare professionals to decrease readmissions, address healthcare disparities, inform biomedical ethics decisions, and improve the patient experience.

AdventHealthPress.com

19-PL-8-01208

Hear more from

MARK HERTLING

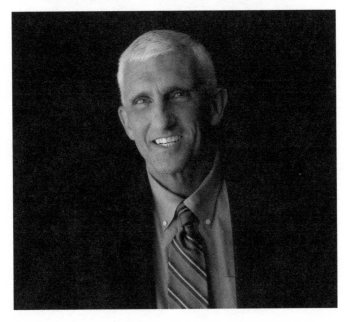

MARK HERTLING SPEAKS ON MANY

TOPICS INCLUDING:

- **Leadership Lessons:** Character, Presence, and Intellect
- **What the Army Has Learned about Our Nation's Fitness**
- **Obesity as a National Security Concern**
- **Commanding During the Surge:** The 1st Armored Division in Northern Iraq
- **Adventures of a CNN Military Analyst**
- **Be, Know and Do:** The Fundamentals of Leadership

To book Mark Hertling or another speaker for your event, visit:

A d v e n t H e a l t h P r e s s . c o m